REWIRE
YOUR
MINDSET

OWN YOUR THINKING,
CONTROL YOUR ACTIONS,
CHANGE YOUR LIFE!

BRIAN KEANE

RETHINK PRESS

First published in Great Britain in 2019 by Rethink Press
(www.rethinkpress.com)

Contents

Prologue

Anne Lamott once observed that all writers 'are little rivers running into one lake', all contributing to the same big project. I consider myself immensely fortunate to have been influenced by so many incredible people over the years, and without the ideas, philosophies and teachings of the people whose lives have interwoven with mine, this book would have never come to pass.

Any acknowledgement, praise or applause for the writing below should not be directed to me but to those who have had a positive impact on me over the years. Even the negative people I have encountered deserve equal appreciation as every person with whom I have ever come in contact has moulded my personality, character and sense of self over the years.

Truth be told, as you will see from reading *Rewire Your Mindset*, owning the fire from negative people may have an even greater impact on your life than the influence of positive people. Nothing is inherently good or bad, but your perception of it renders it so, and the negativity you encounter can be the fuel to keep you going when times get difficult. On the days when you're tired or don't feel like making an effort, you can use those words as the motivation to get you up and pursuing your dream or goal. When you learn to rewire the way you interpret things by taking responsibility for everything in your life and combining the positive influences with negative fuel, I hope you'll see that you can become virtually unstoppable in your endeavours.

For years, the stories I told myself, my negative self-talk and my unsupportive mind chatter would lead me down a road of self-sabotage, fear and anxiety. Only when I learned to completely own the way I chose to see things was I able to control any change in my life. My mantra – 'own it, control it, change it' – that you'll come across throughout this book was my way of overcoming fear and self-sabotage. For years, I made too many decisions out of fear and worry about the opinions of others.

There is nothing special about me; the only difference between us is that I may be a couple of steps ahead of you in my way of thinking. What I do know, though, is that smart people learn from their mistakes and the smarter ones learn from the mistakes of others. I've woven personal stories from my life into this book to help contextualise some of the ideas presented. But I hope that this book serves as a catalyst for building a stronger mindset and fostering the understanding that nothing in your life – your body, your relationships, your job – is going to change until you start making new decisions or seeing things in different ways.

The truth is that there is no such thing as a new idea, and probably there hasn't been an original thought in thousands of years. But I've tried to bring to you some of the ideas that have greatly supported my own life and transformed me from being a victim who blamed the world for all my problems into a stronger version of myself who owned and changed my life. This mindset of mine has led to some external successes, from building an incredibly profitable international fitness business and becoming a best-selling author to running six back-to-back marathons through the Sahara Desert and surviving a gruelling 230km run through the Arctic. Over the years, I've also travelled the world as a professional fitness expert, competed in multiple bodybuilding shows and run multiple marathons and ultramarathons, but it's the inward success I have achieved that I truly value. I would never have been able to achieve any outward success if I wasn't inwardly in control of what I thought, did or said, and I had to learn to do all of that.

The aim of this book is to help you attain inward success by controlling the way you see situations, conditioning yourself to feel fear and do the things you fear anyway, learning how to avoid self-sabotage, and applying strategies such as creating the right habits and using the full power of the compound effect to secure your goals. It's this inward success that leads us to any subjective outward achievement, and the principles in this book go through it all. I wasn't born with any of these capabilities, and I had to develop them through struggle, sacrifice and self-awareness. Although your goals may be completely different from mine, I hope this book serves as a blueprint for ceasing being a victim and taking responsibility for everything that happens to you.

As I'll discuss in later chapters, success is relative; you might be looking to build enough confidence to finally talk to that person you fancy or eliminate self-sabotage when it comes to your eating and training so that you can look the way you want to look. You might even be trying to rewire your mindset so that you feel fear and do the things you're afraid of anyway. Different sections of the book will resonate with you in different ways. The key is not to stop at reading. Once something resonates with you, be sure to make a note of it and follow it up with the action steps that take you closer to your end goal, whatever that is.

My hope for this book is that you exactly get what you need from it. There is an old saying (commonly attributed to the Theosophists) that 'the teacher will appear when the student is ready'. I've had multiple teachers over the years who just seem to appear at the right time – some in the form of books, videos or podcasts, and others in the form of mentors; regardless, all have moulded and shaped my life over the years. Together they helped me to build a mindset that enabled me to achieve whatever I set out to achieve. Remember, such a mindset was built; I wasn't born with it. If a person has ever done what you want to do, it's proof that you can do it too. I hope you use this book the same way that I learned from my teachers. Everything you need to rewire your mindset is in the following pages. Enjoy.

Introduction

'Don't let your own biggest enemy live between your two ears.'
— Laird Hamilton

It was just before midnight on 20 February 2019 in the Arctic, and at -38°C it was bitterly cold. I was 70 km from the Arctic Circle, where I intended to finish a gruelling 230km run through one of the harshest environments on the planet.

My Achilles tendon had been throbbing for several hours. A few days later, I would learn that I tore it 86 km from the finishing line, but for now, I was running on pure adrenaline combined with some painkillers which a member of the local indigenous Sami people had given me.

As I struggled to make it to the finishing line, the mantra that I had often repeated to my four-year-old daughter resounded in my mind: 'If you say you're going to do something, you just go and do it.' With that in mind, I kept moving.

This wasn't always my attitude, though. For a long time in my life, I had done the complete opposite. I would talk about how I was going to do something but never did it. After university, I had plans of starting my own business. Instead, when things got difficult, I went back to the comfort of my old job. In my early twenties, I said I would train for a bodybuilding show. Then, the thought of being on stage in front of thousands of people terrified me, and I dropped the idea. After that, I told everybody how I would run a marathon, but the thought of all the hours of training and hard work put me off, so I dropped that idea too. I had done this over and over again until it had become the foundation on which my life was built.

There was a time when the pain of running through the Arctic with a torn Achilles would have been too much for me. It probably would have even been under-standable to quit there and then.

Nonetheless, this isn't a story about how to run with a torn Achilles or even one about how to survive harsh physical environments; it's a story about taking owner-ship and responsibility for everything in your life – the good, the bad and the ugly. Every failed relationship, every missed job opportunity, every unsupportive diet have all led you to where you are right now, and we're going to use those obstacles as the stepping stones to get you where you want to be. The Arctic ultramarathon was a pivotal test of my mindset. Were all the years of hard work and rewiring my mindset going to pay off when push came to shove, or would I quit as I always had when things became too difficult? That was the pertinent question.

My story

I was born to two working parents and grew up on a farm in the West of Ireland. My family consisted of just my mum, my dad, my little sister and me. Although we didn't have an overabundance of money growing up, we didn't want for anything. Every Christmas or birthday, we got what we asked for (within reason). Despite both my parents working, my sister and I saw our mum every single evening. She always came home after a hard day at work and made food for the both of us and helped us with our homework. My father was gone most of the time. As he worked in the civil service and was heavily involved in local projects, we didn't see him often during the week.

Now that I'm a father, I can see a lot of my parents' personality traits in myself. I got the ability to see the bright side in nearly every situation from my mum. Even though she could be having the worst day, one would have never known it. Also, I admired how she found the time and energy to be with my sister and me even after a nine-hour day and two-hour commute. I feel my ability to work hard and my determination come from my dad. The way he lived his life taught me valuable lessons. Seeing him work nearly every single hour of nearly every day showed me first-hand what one needs to do to be successful in any area of life.

Growing up, I didn't do particularly well in high school and I didn't thrive in traditional education until I got to university. My teenage years were spent playing sport, hooking up with girls and just having a good time. I got into an occasional fistfight when somebody challenged me, but apart from that I was a pretty mellow adolescent.

I graduated high school at seventeen, went straight to university, and secured an undergraduate degree in business and a postgraduate degree in primary school teaching. By the age of twenty-two, I had two degrees to my credit, was living in London and had just landed my first teaching job. It felt like all my hard work over the years was starting to pay off. Yet, every now and again, certain unfulfilled dreams of mine would surface – starting my own business, writing a book, running marathons, participating in bodybuilding shows. But as quickly as they surfaced, I would push them down again and convince myself that they were unrealistic, too difficult or downright unachievable. I would tell myself the story that these were things that other people did, not people like me. My mindset was weak.

It was the worst kind of weakness, as I didn't even acknowledge it as a weakness. My thoughts were on autopilot, and I never questioned whether they were serving me well. At that stage in my life and for the next two years, I was as far as humanly possible from being somebody who could run marathons in the Sahara or the Arctic. At the time, I hated my job, didn't have any meaningful relationships and thought life was just something that happened *to* me and not something that happened *for* me.

My mindset had become weak from years of putting myself down and giving too much weight to the opinions of others, and I would have never believed that I could change my mindset. Over the years, I learned to transform my fear, self-sabotaging and negative self-talk to confidence, desire and, most importantly, belief. I want this book to be your shortcut on your journey of rewiring your mindset. It took me over seven years to change mine, but as the famous quote by Brendan Mull goes, 'Smart people learn from their mistakes; the really sharp ones learn from the mistakes of others.'

The past few years were characterised by a constant struggle to rewire my mindset so that my own biggest enemy didn't live between my two ears anymore. I decided several years ago that I had harboured my enemy long enough and it was time for it to move out. This enemy was like a horrible roommate who never went away. It had taken up residence in my mind, and I had fed it, clothed it and looked after it for so long. Why would it ever want to leave?

We all have some version of that enemy in our heads. It is that voice telling you that you're not smart enough, you're not attractive enough, you're simply not good enough. It may wear a mask of fear and tell you really persuasive stories about all the bad things that could happen to you if you pursue that new job, approach that person to whom you're attracted or set foot in that gym, but that's all they are – stories.

My quest to quieten that voice has led to the writing of this book. The journey involved considerable trial, error and experimenting with my own life. The following chapters are a blueprint for how to rewire your mindset so that your journey doesn't take seven years as mine did.

If you're reading this book, there is some area of your life that you feel needs support or improvement. That's a good thing. You can't change anything until you first identify the problem. Nobody was stopping me from living the life I wanted – except me! Admitting to myself that my own thinking was letting me down was the start of my journey. That journey has led to starting my own business, travelling the world as a professional fitness model, becoming a best-selling author, and becoming a father, ultra-endurance athlete and professional speaker. The transformation starts with a theme you will find recurring in this book: owning and taking responsibility for all the shortcomings or failures in your life to this point.

I grew up watching superheroes like Batman, Spiderman and Superman – heroes who always came to save the day in the end. But my life wasn't a comic book or a movie, and neither is yours. This is real life, and the day I realised nobody was coming to save me was the day I decided it was up to me to change things. I needed to find a way to make myself mentally stronger so that I could handle all the difficulties life threw at me. I needed to become my own hero. This book challenges you to become yours.

Be your own hero

One of my mentors once asked me, 'Who's your hero?'
I instinctively replied, 'My mum', for some of the reasons mentioned earlier but for countless others as well.
As my mentor contemplated my answer, I asked, 'Why, who's your hero?' To my surprise, without skipping a beat, he answered:

> My future self. You see, it's great to have
> heroes in your life. It may be your mum, your
> dad, your brother, your sister, even a teacher
> or a mentor, but if you really want to become
> the best version of yourself, your hero needs
> to be you, but ten years from now ... You see,
> you never truly meet your hero. In ten years,
> I'll have become the person my forty-year-old
> self needed. At fifty, I'll have become the person my forty-year-old self needed, and so on.
> Do you understand what I'm saying?

I understood his message, loud and clear. At the time, though, my twenty-four-year-old self grappled with so many problems, struggles and confidence issues that I could barely even picture what the 'hero me in ten years' would even look like. I had the toxic habit of not believing that I could attain the things I truly desired, so even when good things came into my life, I would inevitably push them away through various methods of self-sabotage.

The above conversation with my mentor opened my eyes to the massive limitations in my thinking. I had been asked about my heroes before, but then I realised I had been seeing the hero subject incorrectly. The realisation didn't make my first answer any less true, but I learned I had only been seeing one piece of the puzzle. If I was going to make myself better, my hero needed to become me, but in ten years. It hasn't been quite ten years since my mentor first asked the question, but at this point it has been pretty close. The first thing my hero needed to do was get rid of that damned enemy between his two ears, so that was what I worked on first.

Challenges

I learned that every time I undertook a challenge, such as running a marathon, or even engaged in an uncomfortable conversation with loved ones or work colleagues, my life improved, and the enemy in my head quietened. It didn't appreciate me getting up at 5am to go to the gym, facing the reality that I was choosing work commitments over my family or questioning my self-created limitations.

It was comfortable when I lived life on autopilot, never challenging my beliefs or questioning my physical limits and unsupportive behaviour. It was comfortable being comfortable, and to quieten it I needed to become comfortable being uncomfortable.

In February 2019, as I battled fatigue and pain during my run through the Arctic at -38°C, with a torn Achilles tendon, my inner enemy was back, louder than ever, although I had spent the last four years keeping it quiet.

First, its voice started as a little whisper: 'You need to quit.' It progressively grew louder with each step: 'You're going to die. Nobody will mind that you didn't finish. You have a torn Achilles, for God's sake. Just quit now. You know you want to. You've come far enough. You're done. Just quit.'

The problem with the voice was that it sounded immensely persuasive when telling me that, 'Nobody will judge you for stopping now' or 'Who else could have come this far?' or 'You should be so proud' or '160 km is far enough, well done'.

For so long, that hypnotic voice had convinced me it was right, and I had fought to overcome it. Now, it had the perfect opportunity to come back into my life; but I knew if it did, it wouldn't go away again easily. I countered the voice saying, 'Quit, you've come far enough' with 'Shut the f*ck up! I'm finishing this run whether you're with me or not. I didn't come this far only to come this far.' Then, I put my left foot in front of my right foot and repeated that for the next 70 km.

A part of me died that night in the Arctic, but it was a weak part – the last scintilla of self-doubt, the last whit of unworthiness, the last bit of personal negativity. Less than twenty-four hours later, on 21 February, after running 230 km, I crossed the Arctic Circle and defeated the enemy.

So what had changed? How did something that would have seemed so unrealistic and unachievable once upon a time become a reality? True, I had trained physically for the gruelling challenge, but I had been in decent shape before as well. Also, now I had the finances to fund such a trip, something I could never have done before, but that wasn't the reason either. It wasn't my body or bank account that had changed. It was my mindset.

Although my Achilles tendon throbbed like a pulsing heartbeat and my body shivered uncontrollably if I stopped even for a second, I committed to crossing the Arctic Circle.

That night, the beautiful snow-covered terrain was pitch black except for the reflection of the moon and slight illumination of the northern lights on the ice. There, as I put one foot in front of the other, I reflected on my life to that point. I didn't feel like it was the end, but I knew that the temptation to lie down in the snow and just let the pain wash over me was real. Years ago, when things had got difficult, that had been exactly what I had done – I quit, buried my head in the sand (or snow, in this case) and ignored the problem or figuratively lay down and died (gave up). Not that night. That night, I kept moving forward.

With every step, my Achilles tendon radiated pain through my entire body, but it got me one step closer to the end goal. I had run 160 km already, I had 70 km to go, and I wouldn't stop. Hell, I couldn't stop. I had my daughter to get home to. I had a family to see again. I had a message that I needed to share with the world. That message became as clear as the moon that night.

Nobody is born with the mindset to go after the things they want; nobody is born with an internal 'happiness' that supersedes every other thought; nobody is born fearless or with the tools to get through any struggle. You develop all of that over time.

Each of us is born as a blank slate, but our experiences over the years mould how we see the world. In the chapter on 'The Compound Effect', I discuss how a walk down a street in East London seven years ago changed my life forever. That walk was the first time I reflected on why I felt so unhappy, unmotivated and unfulfilled.

At the time, I felt unfulfilled in my work and dragged myself out of bed every morning to get to work because I needed the paycheque. I was unhappy with my personal relationships and isolated myself from the people closest to me because I felt so lost and lonely. Unmotivated in every area of my life, I never believed that I could make any real difference in the world. Any time I did get any attention or praise, I would deflect it because I felt unworthy of receiving it. I would sabotage nearly every area of my life because my mindset was so weak. I knew I wanted to live a different kind of life and needed to rewire my mindset but just didn't know how.

I knew I wanted to travel the world and see places like the Sahara and the Arctic, but I let the story of 'That's what other people do' dictate my actions for far too long. Until my mid-twenties, I never questioned the belief, assuming that everything I thought was right. Why would I think it otherwise? I couldn't separate facts from opinions or beliefs, and I never realised that my thinking was the problem, not my circumstances. My mindset was the problem, not my job or relationships.

Throughout the following chapters, I hope you will see all the self-limiting stories that may be holding you back. Different parts of this book will resonate with different people. Some of you may take one or two nuggets of gold that serve as the catalyst for a positive change; others may take the layout of the four quadrants and plug them directly into their current routine, while many may take every single message and strategy and apply them to their own lives wholeheartedly. If you view this book like a gold miner searching for gold, I do not doubt that you will find what you're looking for.

The message contained in the ensuing pages is about looking for the nuggets of gold to improve your mindset so that every decision you make is conscious from this point onwards. You will no longer be making decisions on autopilot or just 'letting things happen to you' – if you want to make a meaningful change in your life, then you've come to the right place.

You may not need to rewire your mindset to run six back-to-back marathons in the Sahara or 230 km through the Arctic, but you may need to build your confidence so that you can go after that job you desire or avoid the self-sabotaging behavioural patterns that stop you from getting into great physical shape. You may have no aspirations to start your own business or become a professional fitness model, but you may need to rewire your focus or lifestyle so that you can finally get the loving relationship and connections you crave.

As mentioned in the prologue, I've used some of my personal experiences to give context to certain ideas throughout the book, but this story isn't about me; it's about helping you see where your mindset needs rewiring. Up until now, you may have seen things like *failure* and *fear* as bad. That's not the truth. That's just a perspective and an opinion. By the end of the book, I hope that you, as the reader, will start to rewire your mindset and use failure and all the things that once held you back as the stepping stones to your future success. Every failed diet or bad relationship or missed job opportunity is feedback on how you can improve in the future.

Every fear you harbour, be it going after a promotion or raise, approaching someone at a bar, or worrying what people will say about the choices you make, will serve you if you learn to control it. Too much fear can paralyse you, but in the right amount it can be the most supportive emotion you'll ever connect with, provided you learn to channel it correctly.

In the coming chapters, you will see how focusing on small, seemingly insignificant changes can have a massive impact on your life in the long term. One of the most quoted lines from my podcast *The Brian Keane Podcast* is 'Tell me what you do every day, and I'll tell you where you'll be in a year'. This quote highlights the power of habits and the importance of what you do every day. As one of my mentors told me, 'You don't decide your future; you decide your habits, and your habits decide your future'.

We'll be combining this idea with the significance of 'the compound effect' and how even the most difficult things become considerably easier over time. Understanding at a visceral level that difficult times are going to pass will make it so much easier to stay on course and not go off track.

On that note, let's come to terms with the fact that things *will* get difficult. Taking ownership of every decision you've made up until now (good and bad) is hard. Nobody wants to admit their shortcomings, failures or mistakes – especially me – but knowing that *owning it* is the key to dealing with anxiety, stress and insecurities makes the philosophy considerably easier to adopt. As you'll learn very soon, when you own something, you can control it, and when you control it, you can change it. This book will challenge some of your long-held opinions about yourself, and sections such as 'The purple polar bear' are going to make uncomfortable reading if you struggle with negativity or other people's opinions of you. Still, by the end of this book, you're going to be so comfortable being uncomfortable that you might even go back and reread it from the start and see what resonates with you the second time around.

This book will take you on a journey from acknowledging any self-limiting stories that you've created to building a specific plan for what you need to do to be successful in all the four quadrants of your life (health, wealth, love and fulfilment). However, before we get into any of that, let's delve into what is the ultimate end goal for nearly all of us. Some use different words to describe it – peace, joyfulness, fulfilment, contentment. Keeping it simple, I just call it 'happiness'.

I

Rewire Your Happiness

'Happiness is not something readymade. It comes from your own actions.'
— Dalai Lama

The term *happiness* is tricky as it means different things to different people. Even so, I choose to use the term here because that's what we're all seeking in some form at the end of the day. Happiness is the sea into which all the other rivers flow. Getting a new job, transforming your body and finding the love of your life are all examples of these rivers, and that's why I have chosen to start this book with a chapter on happiness.

Everything you are about to read is going to flow into the same ending. The way you interpret the world and the actions you take will dictate the course of your life from this point forward. As mentioned above, you may use another term to describe happiness, be it 'peace', 'fulfilment' or something else, but all of them pertain to the same feeling. It's the sense that nothing is missing at the moment.

If you've picked up this book, you may feel some area of your life needs improvement, and my goal is to give you the tools required to address that. I consider myself lucky for not always having possessed a strong mindset. I made bad choices regarding the people I spent time with, the foods I ate and the stories I told myself. Had I been naturally blessed with a strong mindset, I never would have asked the questions or taken the actions that actually made me mentally and physically stronger. Over the course of reading this book, I want you to come to the understanding that every failure or perceived failure you've had in your life up until this point is the seed for your future success. Every failed diet, every co-dependent relationship, every hour spent doing a job you despised – all of those experiences will be the seeds for your future success.

Seeds of past failure bear fruits of future success

If I had loved my first job, married my college sweetheart and never left the little village where I grew up, I wouldn't have become the person I needed to be, and you would not be reading this book. All human potential is born out of struggle and failure. You may have been told that struggle and failure are undesirable, but I'm here to tell you the complete opposite. Your struggles and failures up until this point are the foundational pillars upon which the life you dream of is going to be built! I'm not saying that attaining your dream life is going to be easy. This isn't a wishy-washy

'Dream it, hope for it, and it will manifest itself in your life' kind of book; rather, this is a 'Dream it, hope for it, work your freaking ass off, and it will manifest itself in your life' kind of book.

You will see in the coming chapters that once you get your figurative ladder up against the right wall – once you start going after what you truly want – working hard will not feel as difficult as you may have thought and your past failures will serve as the floor on which that ladder is planted.

I'm grateful for every failure in my life as each of them has taught me what *not* to do next time. I grew up in a working-class family and went broke three times trying to start my own business, so my knowledge of money and how it worked was pretty limited. Yet, those circumstances and experiences allowed me to acquire the skills to make money and invest better as an adult. Now I wake up every day feeling blessed in that area of my life.

Starting my own business was a similar experience. Having always struggled with authority, as I grew older I started to lose faith in people older and more senior than me. This led me on the journey of creating my own business. My business has served thousands of people with programmes, courses and seminars over the years, which allows me to 'tap dance to work' every day, as the billionaire investor Warren Buffett puts it.

My relationships took the same route. The realisation that I was becoming weaker when I continued to stay in the wrong relationship – business, romantic or personal – led me to get more comfortable with difficult conversations, which allowed me to become a better partner, father and son.

I owe my mental and physical well-being to having lived on the other end of the spectrum for much of my early life. During my teenage years, I was physically sick and battled bouts of depression and contemplations of suicide. Those dark moments made me focus on my mental and physical health. Currently, I am probably the happiest person on the planet and have a family, job and life that I wouldn't trade for anything. Nevertheless, all that was born out of darkness. As the great psychiatrist Carl Jung said, 'Your branches can't reach to heaven if your roots don't go down to hell.'[1] I had to deal with the lows, but now I live a life of constant highs because of it.

Every issue, problem or setback in your life is going to make you stronger, tougher and happier if you decide not to let it break you and turn it into a positive.

Things you know, things you don't know, and things you don't know that you don't know

I discuss goal setting and hitting targets later on, but at the end of the day, happiness is the main metric of success for most people. You can have the best body in the world, the nicest car, the coolest clothes, the

---

1   C G Jung (1959) *Aion: Researches into the Phenomenology of the Self: Collected works of C G Jung.* London: Routledge.

prettiest wife or the most handsome husband, but despite having all that, if you're still unhappy, then none of those things really make you feel any better. As you'll see in the following chapters, I have learned this from personal experience because I have lived through it.

Sometimes you need to be able to identify a problem before finding a solution for it. For example, if you go to a doctor with high cholesterol, the doctor will prescribe you some medicine to help with the ailment. But what if you don't know you have a problem in the first place? That was my issue. I didn't think there was anything wrong with my thinking.

Let's take a step back before I continue with this theme. There are only three broad categories of problems – the things we know, the things we don't know and the things we don't know that we don't know. The things we don't know that we don't know are silent killers.

The things you know are pretty straightforward. As you know you have a problem, you can deal with it accordingly if you want to.

The things you don't know are a little more problematic but not critical. Once you realise you have a problem or issue, then you can try and find someone or something that can fix it.

The things you don't know that you don't know do all the damage. That's what happened to me when I came up with the 'I'll be happy when' fallacy. It was my automatic way of thinking, like my thoughts were on autopilot. I never questioned them. I never realised that this way of thinking was making me unhappy in so many areas of my life. I didn't know that I didn't know the correct path to happiness, so I couldn't start walking down the path.

I would tell myself stories like, 'I'll be happy when I graduate from college', 'I'll be happy when I get my first job' and 'I'll be happy when I get that pay raise', never realising that if I am not happy on the journey, I'm not going to be happy when I arrive at my destination.

It took me years to come to the understanding that happiness is a choice I need to make and a skill I need to develop. One can do this by putting one's ladder up against the right wall and regularly asking oneself, 'Am I enjoying this climb? Am I enjoying this process?'

Having your ladder against the right wall means that you have total clarity about your end goal. As you'll see in the 'Rewire Your Goal Setting' chapter, you cannot hit a target you cannot see. When you are crystal clear about the relationship you want, the body you want, the job you want or anything else you want, that's getting your ladder up against the right wall.

If you find yourself regularly questioning your climb, wondering whether it's the right kind of suffering that makes you better or gets you closer to your end goal, then it's probably time you consider whether your ladder is up against the right wall in the first place.

Thinking you're stuck in some area of your life is like self-imposed imprisonment in most cases. You think you can't make a change because you have invested too much time, money or energy into a particular job, relationship or fitness programme and there's too much to lose if you change the direction now. I'm here to tell you that this is not true. It is not a fact but merely an opinion. In most cases, facts cannot be changed. Opinions can be. Unfortunately, so many of us often confuse the two.

Confusing opinions for facts

'Everything we see is a perspective, not a fact;
everything we hear is an opinion, not a truth.'
— Marcus Aurelius

If you jump out of a ten-storey building, you'll go splat when you hit the ground, owing to the law of gravity. That's a fact. When you tell yourself you can't lose weight or you aren't smart enough for a job or you're not attractive enough for a person, that's an opinion. When you learn to distinguish facts from opinions, you will see how quickly things begin to change, and your mind starts to open to new ideas.

I can't give you the exact recipe for happiness, but I can give you some ingredients of misery.

One ingredient of misery is never questioning your self-limiting story. I did this for most of my early twenties. When I was looking to start my own business, I knew I wanted to create something that helped and served people on a grand scale, but my self-limiting story told me that I wasn't good enough or smart enough and that starting a business was something 'other people' did.

If you have ever uttered the words 'Oh, I can never do that' to yourself, then you know exactly what I'm talking about. 'I can never do that' is an opinion, not a fact. You can't change facts, but you can change opinions by taking different actions. Do not confuse the two.

Another ingredient of misery is climbing to the top of the ladder and realising it's against the wrong wall. I had this experience when I was working full time as a primary school teacher. I spent five years studying to become a teacher – four years to secure an honours degree, one year for a postgraduate degree – and then I worked hard to get my first job, only to realise that I didn't enjoy it nearly as much as I thought I would. In fact, I hated my first teaching job, and although I grew to enjoy it after a few years, it never felt like what I was meant to do. Later in this chapter, you will see that it is better to be at the bottom of the ladder against the right wall (your job, your fitness, your relationships, among others) than to be nearly at the top of the ladder against the wrong wall.

When it comes to the ingredients of misery, my personal favourite is making decisions based on the opinions of others. In the past, I made decisions based on what everybody else thought I should do concerning what women I should date, what job I should have and how I should be as a person in general. Although it may be the hardest part of rewiring your mindset,

I hope that by the end of the book you'll have all the tools you need to start living life on your terms and not somebody else's.

I worked as a primary school teacher for four years. As I mentioned above, it was a job I enjoyed but never truly loved, and it was always just a job to me: On Fridays, I knew I was going to be off the coming weekend; and on Monday mornings, I knew I had to go back to work. I would regularly get 'Friday euphoria' – the high that comes before the weekend – and 'Sunday blues' – the low that comes at the end of the weekend.

When I first set up my personal training business, one of my metrics of success I set for myself was not to feel that way anymore. I calculated that I felt 'low' at least forty weeks a year, purely for work-related reasons.

I lived for weekends and vacations, which led to a hollow feeling when I thought about my job. Then, one day after Easter break, as I was preparing for a lesson on Pablo Picasso, I came across a philosophy called 'Picasso's dichotomy' (although Picasso himself didn't invent it), which I still regularly refer to several years later. If you're unfamiliar with the term 'dichotomy' as I was, it means a division or contrast between two things that are represented as being opposed or entirely different.

The philosophy is as follows:

Never permit a dichotomy to rule your life, a
dichotomy in which you hate what you do
so you can have pleasure in your spare time.

> Look for a situation in which your work will
> give you as much happiness as your spare
> time.[2]

I didn't hate my job, but I didn't love it either. Therefore, something had to change. One of the most famous lines from the book *The Alchemist* by Paulo Coelho is: 'When you want something, all the universe conspires in helping you achieve it', and that was how it was starting to feel for me.[3]

When you start to see things differently, you start noticing opportunities that you didn't see before. At the time, my seed of change had been sown. I realised that I was living in a dichotomy and needed to make a change.

Eight years later, I now never pay attention to what day it is. Work and play have merged into one. If I take off from work completely for a day, I itch to get back to it the following morning. At one stage in my life, being in such a place was only a dream and a vision, but that's how it all starts. You may love your job, but you may be struggling with your weight; or you may be in great shape, but you may have trouble with romantic relationships. Being clear about what exactly you want is the first step.

Regardless of your internal belief system, and

---

2   Dennis Wholey (1986) *Are You Happy?: Some answers to the most important question in your life.* Boston, MA: Houghton Mifflin Harcourt, p94.

3   Paulo Coelho (1989) *The Alchemist*. New York: HarperCollins.

whatever your goal is, as the saying goes – 'If you can see it in your mind, you can hold it in your hand'. It all starts with a vision.

I would advise anyone in a similar situation to the one I found myself in to follow their intellectual curiosity over other people's expectations. Teaching primary school was and still is a great job, with decent pay, good holidays and adequate respectability, but it wasn't what I loved – it wasn't the kind of work that made me jump out of bed every morning with enthusiasm.

Having said that, I'm still a teacher to a large extent. The books I write, the podcasts and videos I make, and the speaking I do are all teaching, just in the areas of life about which I'm more passionate and for which I have a stronger calling.

When your curiosity leads you to a place where society wants you to go, you'll get paid extremely well for it. I was happier making £20,000 a year as a personal trainer than £40,000 a year as a teacher. Fortunately, I make considerably more now, but for personal training the happiness factor was a 10/10 then and still is now. Once your basic needs of food, clothing and shelter are covered, money doesn't make you happier; instead, it just allows you to buy more stuff.

I found happiness when I started to lose myself in the service of others, which is exactly what I hope to achieve with this book. Just because you can't see happiness right now doesn't mean it can't happen in the future. As mentioned above, there are things you know, things you don't know, and things you don't know that you don't know. My goal is to get you to ask the questions that allow you to see things from a different angle. If your reflex was 'I don't know what my gift or talent is' – or worse, 'I have no gift or talent' – by the time you've finished this book I hope you will see that is just a story you've told yourself up until now.

Confucius captured the idea at its best when he preached, 'He who said he can and he who said he can't are both usually right'.[4] As soon as you tell your-self you have no talents or gifts, your mind will close off and your confirmation bias – the cognitive bias that shuts off all other possibilities of disconfirming evidence – will kick in, and you'll be 'right'. A mentor of mine once told me that one could be happy or one could be right, but one couldn't always be both. Still, if you rewire your mindset and open up your mind to the possibility that you have something bigger than yourself to offer the world, then you start to ask better questions. Try the following subtle sentence change the next time you think you can't do something: When your head says, 'I can't do it', switch the words to 'How can I do it?' and pay attention to the thoughts that begin to appear and see how your mind starts to open up to other possibilities.

Someone once told me, 'Smart people have great answers; geniuses have great questions'. Therefore, following his advice, 'How can I serve the world?' or

---

4   From Confucius' *The Analects*.

'What talents do I possess that other people need?' are good questions to ask yourself.

By the way, what one wants to do is relative. For some, it's changing the world through their words and actions, like Mother Teresa, Martin Luther King Jr or Gandhi. For others, it's being an inspiration for those around them – maintaining a healthy lifestyle or being a great parent, partner, son or daughter. Finding what is important to you and the things that make you feel happy and fulfilled is the key.

For most of my life, I lived by the 'I can't' thought process. I kept telling myself that 'I can't start my own business', 'I can't become a professional fitness model', 'I can't compete as a bodybuilder' and 'I can't run six back-to-back marathons through the Sahara', which were all self-limiting belief systems I once held. These were all former fears that I had to overcome, but for a long time my 'I can't' thought process was automatic.

A very funny thing happens when you start to question such belief systems: You realise that they're all based on fear and that you're letting your fear dictate your decisions and actions. My favourite acronym for FEAR is False Evidence Appearing Real, and as soon as I started to question why I couldn't do the things that I wanted to do, I realised I had a belief system grounded in fear, and that was what held me back.

The first leap I made in my life was going from being a full-time primary school teacher to starting my own business as a personal trainer. I juggled both jobs for two years, and although I was tired, I knew deep down that my second job – my 'side hustle' – was what I really wanted to do. The real catalyst of change, however, came after reading a book called *Rich Dad Poor Dad* by Robert Kiyosaki.[5]

Rich Dad Poor Dad is about a boy who has two dads: One is his real dad, and the other is his best friend's dad. One is a well-educated teacher with a master's degree, and the other is a high school dropout. One is always worrying about paying bills and never seems to have enough money, and the other is buying real estate and businesses and becoming one of the richest men in the country. The narrative set-up seemed obvious to me – the educated graduate was surely the rich dad. Alas, no. It was actually the opposite, and as trivial as that fact may be, it served to bring about a complete paradigm shift in me.

I had grown up to believe that to be 'successful', one had to go to college, get a degree, locate a good job, find a partner, buy a house, get married, have kids, retire at sixty-five, and then travel the world or play golf. Although I never consciously thought about it, my actions were leading me down that path. I often reiterate on my podcast that if you tell me what you do every day, I'll tell you where you'll be in a year. The same goes for five years, ten years, and so on. We are what we repeatedly do. This concept is so powerful that I have dedicated specific chapters called 'The Compound Effect' and 'Rewire Your Habits' to it in this book.

---

5   R Kiyosaki (1997) *Rich Dad Poor Dad*. Plata Publishing.

Before I made the leap, I was just kind of going along on autopilot, living life in a pre-programmed way, never questioning anything. I was riding the horse of my habits but had no control of the direction it was taking me.

Rich Dad Poor Dad made me question the belief system of working a regular nine-to-five job and sparked the thought, 'What other questions have I not been asking?' prompting me to think deeply about the habits, belief systems and opinions that weren't serving me anymore.

I had read the book in October 2013, and I left my last teaching job two months later. The book also set me on a path of cutting my learning curve through reading more books and learning from others' mistakes as well as my own.

Getting my business off the ground was difficult. I had to move back in with my parents. At the time, I was driving my sister's twenty-year-old Toyota Yaris. I remember my friends making fun of me because the car was nearly as old as I was! I had moved from London back to Ireland and had to go on welfare for several months before I could get any clients. Admittedly, at the time, I was embarrassed (again caring about the opinions of others – a key ingredient of misery or anxiety), but I knew my ladder was against the right wall. I had to keep telling myself that it was better to be at the bottom of the ladder against the right wall that halfway up the ladder against the wrong wall.

At the time, working in a gym and helping people

transform their bodies (and mindsets in a lot of cases) were things I would have done for free. After a few months, I started getting paid for it. Fast forward eight years and my business currently serves thousands of people every year in an online capacity with programmes and courses. My first book *The Fitness Mindset* became an international bestseller, and I get to travel all over the world to speak or attend different events that help people become stronger versions of themselves. I'm not saying this out of ego or bravado. Pride always comes before the fall, but you're also always your own best example. Remember, if you can see it in your mind, apply the action steps daily, visualise it clearly and work hard for it, you can achieve virtually anything!

After that, it's about building the confidence to do it again and again.

Confidence

I like to think of confidence as the legs of a table; the more legs a table has, the sturdier and stronger it becomes. Confidence comes from saying you're going to do something and then going out and actually doing it. One of the reasons I love fitness so much is that it's an incredible metaphor for how one does anything in life. If you join a gym, you don't transform overnight from unfit and overweight or weak and skinny to strong, lean and muscular. But, if you consistently go to the gym and exercise, each workout gets a little easier than the one before; you get a little better and you become stronger, leaner or fitter over time.

Before I elaborate on confidence, I want to discuss the 'I'll be happy when' fallacy, which I mentioned earlier. This one misconception can take all the legs away from a table in one fell swoop.

One of the misconceptions people have about fitness or any other area of life is the 'I'll be happy when' fallacy – 'I'll be happy when I'm at this weight or fit into that dress or t-shirt'. It's having a picture in your mind of what you want to look like or the car you want to drive or the position you want to hold, all the while thinking that reaching your goals is going to make you feel better about yourself. But this just isn't true.

I hate to be the one to break it to you, but attaining your goals will not make you happy or fulfilled. Yes, those things are all incredible to have, and you should have the ambition to go after them if that's what you desire. But the process of becoming who you have to become to achieve your desires in the first place is where real fulfilment lies. That's why the process of setting your goals is so important.

If you're chasing a number on the weighing scale or a number in your bank account, then every time you hit that number your figurative bar moves, and you'll want more.

Yes, you may enjoy a momentary feeling of happiness or fulfilment, having hit your target. Nevertheless, if those numbers are your metrics of success, once the initial good feeling of having achieved your goal wears off you will set the next goal, going back to feeling the same way you did on day one. I've set goals and gone back to setting higher targets, having achieved my original goal time and time again. As Benjamin Franklin said, 'Experience keeps a dear school, but a fool will learn in no other'. I had to learn it the hard way, but you definitely don't need to learn it that way.

What if I tell you instead of focusing just on your end goal to focus on each step of the journey or rung of the ladder? Yes, look to the top and keep your end goal in mind, but focus on putting one foot in front of the other while stopping regularly to ask the question, 'Am I enjoying the process?' If the answer is most often positive, then keep climbing. If not, then it's time to re-evaluate things.

As I mentioned, confidence comes from saying you are going to hit a target or achieve a goal and then doing it. The more you do that, the more figurative legs you'll add to your table. All the same, if you don't fix this one reframe on confidence, then every time you hit your target, that hollow feeling will accompany it, and all those legs can shatter in one fell swoop. If you've ever witnessed a 'successful' person encounter a huge failure and be figuratively broken by it, the downfall normally would have come from that one swoop. There's a reason people use the expression 'the world comes crashing down' when describing an epic failure. The same thing happens when too much weight is put on a table held up by wobbly legs: it breaks and comes crashing down.

Yes, I've done it! Uh... Now what?

Have you ever seen somebody close to you achieve a really big goal they set for themselves? They've been working towards it for weeks, months or even years, and now they've hit it. In a lot of cases, one of two things happens after they reach their goal. One is negative; the other is positive.

They either realise all their hard work was for nothing and feel hollow after it (ladder-against-the-wrong-wall syndrome), or they seem completely transformed, having overcome all their limitations, with a new glow about them – an overriding, infectious and radiating confidence. What factors lead to each outcome?

The first one is pretty obvious: If you're climbing a ladder against the wrong wall, you will know deep down that you're chasing the wrong things, but you ignore it and keep going. Then, you're going to feel hollow when you actually reach the top.

The second one is much more interesting. If you focus on becoming the person you need to be to achieve a specific goal, then the actual goal is just one more step on the ladder.

I've experienced both, and both circumstances transformed me in very different ways.

Ladder against the wrong wall – Fitness Model World Championships

In 2015, I finished eighth in the World Fitness Model Championships held in Las Vegas. I had spent six months preparing for the competition, eating six meals a day, counting my macronutrient and calorie intake, training several hours a day and pushing my body to its limits daily.

At that point in my life, I was completely out of balance. I stopped spending time with my friends and family because it interfered with my training or meal preparation. My business wasn't growing as quickly as I would have liked since I was overworked and tired all the time and putting more effort and energy into my training than my clients.

True, I was getting bigger and leaner, and I finished in the top ten at the World Championships. Yet, as soon as the show ended, I felt hollow. For the first time in about six months, I was able to evaluate my life from a 30,000-foot bird's eye view. Yes, I had only 5% body fat and was lean and muscular, but I was lonely, unhappy and unfulfilled.

I realised I had been blinded by ambition, though not for the first time in my life. I had just achieved my goal of becoming one of the top fitness model competitors in the world, but I had no one to share it with. Nonetheless, the truth is that I wouldn't trade that experience for anything. The seed for the concept of the four quadrants that I discuss in the next chapter was first planted here. In hindsight, though, it didn't have to be this way.

If I had stopped and asked myself the question, 'Am I enjoying this process?' at any stage over those six months, I would have seen how unbalanced my life had become and I'd have been able to course correct. Now, I ask that question regularly in everything that I do. Concerning any work I do, any training programme I follow, any relationship I'm in (business, romantic or otherwise), I ask myself two simple questions:

1. Is this helping with the end goal?
2. Am I enjoying the process?

The power of the above two questions has helped me more than anything else with my daily happiness and fulfilment levels. Try it. Regardless of the area of your life that you are trying to improve right now, ask yourself the two simple questions.

Regarding the first question, let's look at your diet, for example. If you are trying to lose weight or body fat, is the food you are eating every day helping with your end goal? If you're eating ice cream and cake all day, the answer is probably no. If you're eating broccoli and salad all day, then the answer is probably yes as such a diet will probably help you lose weight. Now, that's when the second question becomes important.

Are you enjoying the process? Even if your desire to lose weight is high, eating salad for all meals is eventually going to become boring and monotonous, and you'll grow to hate it. I don't know anyone on this planet who can do something they absolutely hate every single day of their life. Yes, you may be able to do it for a week, a month, a year or even five years, but eventually, the pain and lack of enjoyability of the process will force you to change, for better or for worse.

In 2015, while participating in the competition, even though my actions led me to my end goal, I never focused on the process. I saw the end goal of the show as my end goal. If I had been smarter, I would have seen it as just one more step on the ladder. I learned from the mistake and adopted a new strategy when I ran six back-to-back marathons in the Sahara in 2018.

Ladder against the right wall – Marathon des Sables

In April 2018, I set myself the goal of completing the Marathon des Sables (MDS), which constituted six back-to-back marathons through the Sahara in Morocco. The race also requires the participants to be self-sufficient as one has to carry all the required food and equipment on one's back during the race. The Sahara is one of the hottest places on earth, making this event unlike any I had ever seen before.

I had heard about the MDS at a conference I attended in the summer of 2017. My friend told me about an intense race he had done in the Sahara. He spoke about people being hooked to intravenous drips due to dehydration, keeping a venom pump within arms' reach in case of being bitten by a snake and running six back-to-back marathons. It sounded insane, and I was hooked to every word that came out of his mouth. I spent the next hour of the conference checking out the MDS website. I signed up for it three months later. At that point in my life, having to run six back-to-back marathons in less than eight months seemed a daunting challenge as I had never even run a single marathon before.

I did my first run the day I signed up. It was a 2km run, and I nearly got sick! Not having run more than 2 km in years, I really started to question my decision. To keep myself accountable, I posted about it across all my social media accounts. Now, there was no pulling out.

I knew training for the marathon was going to require considerable work, but I was committed to not repeating my previous mistake and becoming blinded by the end goal. I needed to focus on the process, not just the result. In training terms, I went from running 2 km a day to 3 km, 5 km, 10 km and then eventually over 20 km, and so on.

Instead of focusing just on the target, I prioritised getting each day right and enjoying the actual process. Every run got me a little bit closer to my end goal, but I regularly stopped and asked myself, 'Am I enjoying the process?' This strategy allowed me to maintain balance in all the other areas of my life. I speak more about MDS in the 'Rewire Fear' chapter, but for now, I would like to say that it serves as a contrast to the

Fitness Model World Championships. In 2015, I only focused on the end goal and never took my head out of the figurative clouds. In 2018, the opposite happened. I knew preparing for the marathon was going to take considerable time, energy and effort, so I decided to just get up earlier than usual to train. I spent more time with my family, friends and inner circle, and my business actually grew during this period. I compartmentalised and set aside a few hours in the morning – 'MDS time' – to train, prepare meals and otherwise get myself ready. Therefore, all the other areas of my life actually improved because I made a conscious choice to ensure my current goal was enhancing my life and not hindering it. This left me feeling focused, happy and fulfilled.

The actions we take lead to the outcomes we receive. We live in a world of cause and effect. Sometimes, we need to go right back to the root cause of a problem to make a change; other times, we have to catch ourselves when we see bad habits creeping in while understanding that this is how the universes works, which is crucial for change or improvement.

Cause and effect

Let me narrate a story I used to tell the clients I trained. A man is standing on the banks of a river. Suddenly, he sees a man caught in the raging current bouncing about on jagged rocks and calling for help. He leaps in, pulls the drowning man to safety, gives him mouth-to-mouth resuscitation, attends to the man's wounds and calls for medical help. As he's catching his breath, he hears two more screams emanating from the river. Again, he jumps in and makes another daring rescue, saving two young women this time. Before he even has a chance to think, he hears four more people calling for help. Soon, the man is exhausted, having rescued victim after victim, but the screams continue. If only he had taken the time and effort to travel a short distance upriver, he could have discovered who was throwing all those people into the water in the first place! He could have saved all his efforts by addressing the problem at the cause rather than its effect.

The story resonated so deeply with me because I was once that guy. I would figuratively put plasters over a bleeding cut and simultaneously bang my head against a wall, all the while wondering why the cut would never heal! In my search for happiness and fulfilment, I bought new cars and nicer clothes and spent countless hours in the gym so that I would feel 'successful'. All plasters over an insecurity.

I've been a long-time subscriber to the idea that your mess becomes your message, and if you don't fix the root problem or control your mindset you just end up plastering over the real problem. You can put someone with their old mindset in the new car or a new body, but they're going to feel the same way if you haven't addressed the root problem. For me, it was placing my happiness and self-worth in external things and repeatedly falling for the 'I'll be happy when' fallacy. One of my mentors used to tell me, 'If you really want to find the root of any problem, ask "why" four times.'

Why do you want to be leaner? Because I want to look better. Why do you want to look better? So that I can feel more confident. Why do you want to feel more confident? To find a boyfriend, girlfriend, husband or wife. Why do you want to find a boyfriend, girlfriend, husband or wife? Because I'm lonely and I'm afraid I'll end up alone. Four whys and you've found the root problem. Fear! As you'll see below, so much of our unhappiness, worries and restlessness are rooted in fear.

You may not need to ask 'why' four times as you may figure out your motivations for pursuing a goal after asking it only once. Sometimes, you may need to ask more than four times, but the principle is the same. You need to get to the root of the problem. If you don't find what is at the root of why you feel a certain way, then you're going to have to tackle the same problem again and again as the guy in the story above and never think of going upstream to fix the source of your problem.

Yes, you can plaster your insecurities with nice clothes, a great body or an awesome car, but once hedonic adaptation (the psychological term for adapting to cool new things) takes place, you're going to go back to feeling the same way as before.

Hedonic adaptation

'It is not the man who has too little, but the man who craves more, that is poor.'
— Seneca

If you're unfamiliar with hedonic adaptation, I would like to use the example of sunrise to explain the concept. If you've ever sat and watched a sunrise, it really is a beautiful sight, and I recommend that you experience it at least once in your life. But, as it happens every single day, we often take it for granted. If you've never seen a sunrise, you probably just thought, 'I should check that out some time', but the thought will pass, and you'll forget about it by tomorrow or even over the next few paragraphs. If a sunrise only happened once every ten or twenty years, though, I bet you would consider planning an entire day, week or possibly even a month around witnessing it.

That's the wicked power of hedonic adaptation, and it leads us to take the most amazing things in our lives for granted: our health, our families, the rights and freedoms we enjoy, and the roof over our heads, among others. The list goes on and on. I could never really connect with the 'at least you have your health' concept until I learned about the concept of hedonic adaptation and the strategy of negative visualisation, a practice I discuss in greater detail in the 'Rewire Your Mental Health' chapter.

Before I continue, it's worth noting that the hedonic adaptation principle works in both directions (thankfully). Those who have suffered a major life trauma can bounce back to their previous happiness baseline after a given period. I also acknowledge that trauma and tragedies outside of a person's control (illness, death of loved ones, political/economic upheaval in the country where a person lives, etc) can seriously affect the person's ability to achieve their goals and be happy, and recovering from trauma can be a separate process from what is in this book. Understanding hedonic adaptation and combining it with negative visualisation may be my two greatest tools for living in a constant state of gratitude. Combining desiring less (at least in the material, plaster-over-a-cut sense) with negative visualisation – the act of thinking about what you currently have and then imagining it being taken away from you – can break hedonic adaptation.

Please note that I'm not saying you shouldn't have nice things. If you love new cars or nice clothes, then go and buy them. I'm just trying to get you to evaluate whether the reason you're buying things is to plaster your insecurities or impress others.

I fall victim to such tendencies as often as anyone else. But my strategy for recognising them consists of asking one simple question, 'Will I want to buy, do or have a certain thing if nobody else is watching or sees me with it?' or put more simply 'If I am stranded on a desert island alone, will I still want to have, do or buy this?'

For example, one of my best friends is obsessed with cars. He loves driving fancy cars, and the faster and more powerful the better. To me, cars are pieces of metal on four pieces of rubber. I have zero emotional attachment to them. If you ask me whether I would buy a fancy, new car if nobody else saw me driving it, the answer would always be no. My friend and I are also opposites regarding working out. He jokes that if I were stranded on a desert island, I'd make a pull-up bar out of a branch and do pull-ups and push-ups every day, and it's true. I love the way exercising makes me feel, and I'll do some form of exercise until the day I die. On the other hand, my friend's exact response when I spoke to him about this part of the book was, 'I'd rather be fat driving my Ferrari around the island'.

I used the above example to present the idea that nothing is right or wrong in itself. Finding out what is important to you, what things you value most and what is on your 'things that make me happy' list is the happiness equivalent to having winning lottery numbers.

Speaking of playing the lottery, arguably the most famous psychological studies on hedonic adaptation have been conducted on lottery winners. In one of these studies, researchers from the University of Massachusetts and Northwestern University asked two separate groups about their levels of happiness: recent winners of the Illinois State Lottery whose prizes ranged from $50,000 to $1 million and recent victims of catastrophic accidents who were now paraplegic or quadriplegic.

In the interviews with the study subjects, the two groups were asked, among other things, to rate the amount of pleasure they derived from small but enjoy-able everyday activities such as chatting with a friend, watching TV, eating breakfast, laughing at a joke or receiving a compliment. When the researchers analysed the results of the study, they found that the recent accident victims reported gaining more happiness from these everyday activities than the lottery winners:

> 'Eventually, the thrill of winning the lottery
> will itself wear off. If all things are judged
> by the extent to which they depart from a
> baseline of past experience, gradually even
> the most positive events will cease to have
> impact as they themselves are absorbed into
> the new baseline against which further events
> are judged.'[6]

Simply put, the above quote means that securing or acquiring anything new in life, like a job, a sweater or a spouse, is exhilarating until we get used to seeing it every day and take it for granted. But maybe the most important thing the research suggests is just how terrible we are at predicting what will make us happy, something psychologists refer to as affective forecasting.

Affective forecasting errors may be particularly common concerning money. Studies show that a

---

6   P Brickman, D Coates, J Janoff-Bulman (1978) 'Lottery Winners and
    Accident Victims: Is happiness relative?', *Journal of Personality and
    Social Psychology*, Vol 36(8): 917.

shorter commute will make you as happy as a 40% pay raise and having more free time can actually make you happier than having more money, and yet most of us, myself included, think that more money is the answer. Some of these errors in forecasting may be partly due to affective forecasting being a relatively new mental trick, one that our brains just haven't had time to perfect yet. On this topic, Dan Gilbert, a Harvard psychologist and the author of *Stumbling on Happiness*, said:

> Modern people take the ability to imagine the future for granted, but it turns out that this is one of our species' most recently acquired abilities – no more than three million years old ... The part of our brain that enables us to think about the future is one of nature's newest inventions, so it isn't surprising that when we try to use this new ability to imagine our futures, we make some rookie errors.[7]

I remember reading Dan Gilbert's book, and it led me down this rabbit hole of understanding hedonic adaptation, happiness and trying to figure out why I was giving so much figurative 'happiness weight' to having things like money and being financially successful.

I spent years trying to build my business to generate X amount of money. I had set a big revenue target several years ago and put the number on the whiteboard

---

7   D Gilbert (2006) *Stumbling on Happiness*. New York: Alfred A Knopf Publishing.

in my office and looked at it every single day. I did everything that would help me hit that target: reading books, listening to podcasts, attending seminars, doing anything and everything that would help me achieve that end goal.

Then, in 2016, I got my year-end financial statement and learned that I had hit my target. Although I had been tracking the revenues, seeing it on the report in black and white brought me huge satisfaction, but only temporarily.

Having hit my target with flying colours, I was proud, but I still felt hollow. For one, I had traded considerable time for financial success, and it had come at the expense of other things – my personal relationships. My daughter had been born in 2015, and her birth had given my life a new directional shift and planted the seed for self-awareness, which would eventually lead me to ask better questions and to set higher standards for the other areas of my life. Regardless, at the time, I couldn't figure out why the win felt so empty.

Then, I did something really stupid. I decided that I didn't feel hollow because I had X amount; it was because I really needed to earn Y amount. Looking back, this was pure insanity; as the saying goes, 'The definition of insanity is doing the same thing over and over again and expecting a different result'. I was trying to save the people in the river instead of going to the riverbank to identify the root of the problem. It took me another twelve months before I realised the root of the problem. I was giving disproportionate weight to things like money and financial success at the expense of the other areas of my life. That's when I really started developing the four-quadrant formula, which is discussed in the next chapter, and I've used it ever since.

Before I delve into the four-quadrant formula, I would like to briefly discuss the disproportionate weight theory – a key concept in developing the four-quadrant formula. To put it simply, allow me to ask a question: Do you think you would be happier if you lived in a hotter country?

If only I lived in a hotter country

If you live in a wet or cold country, the thought 'I'd be so much happier if I just lived in a hotter country' has probably crossed your mind at least once. Yes, living in a hot country definitely has some physiological benefits: the Vitamin D from the sun, the opportunity to engage in outdoor sports, and the ease in organising camping trips and picnics, among others. But think about it a little more deeply. Would you trade all your family and friends for being in the sun all day? Would you trade a job that you absolutely love for one you hate just to go to the beach at the weekends? These are all very valid questions, yet we often give disproportionate weight to one particular thing; in this case, the sun or the weather.

For me, the priority was money. Growing up, although my sister and I never wanted for anything – we always had food in our cupboards, a roof over our head and clothes on our back – money was never in abundance. I learned at an early age that to be 'successful', one needs to make money, and the more money one makes, the more successful one is. Regularly at the dinner table, if someone's name was brought up in conversation, it was quickly followed by their job title and the comments: 'They make great money doing that,' or, 'There's no money in that.' Those conversations shaped the way I saw the world and hardwired my definition of success, although I was unaware of it at the time.

The way you see the world and the thoughts or belief systems you have are a result of your experiences in life up until this point. They're a composition of opinions that have been interwoven together to form a story, a narrative. At the end of the day, they're still opinions, not facts.

One of my ambitions for this book is to get you to see how your story is affecting the way you see the world. As mentioned earlier, you are entitled to your opinions, but you are not entitled to the facts. 'You can't lose weight.' 'You can't earn more money or get a job you love because you're not smart enough.' 'You can't find a loving partner because all the good ones are taken.' None of those is a fact; they're all opinions, stories or excuses that you've formed in your own head. As soon as you stop letting your story dictate the way you see things and own it for what it is, you can control it; and when you control it, you can change it.

Don't plant apple seeds and expect oranges to grow

I consider myself fortunate, for I can become very focused when I'm trying to achieve a goal. The tendency has been to my detriment at times, but it has served me for the most part. When I was training for a bodybuilding show, that was all I worked towards. I didn't go out drinking with friends, I didn't socialise at restaurants, nothing. I ate, breathed and slept bodybuilding.

While building my business, I did the same, although I added working out, which I used to help me de-stress. Otherwise, I ate, worked, consumed business information, slept and repeated that every single day.

Such monomaniacal focus can be helpful from an external viewpoint, but I always think back about it as 'outward success fuelled by inner turmoil' because my mind never shuts off. I walked around in nice clothes, drove a new car and had a thriving business but at the expense of nearly everything else in my life. I had poor relationships with the people closest to me. My health, particularly my mental health, was the worst it had ever been, and I would regularly have sleepless nights, worrying about competitors, wondering if I was growing and scaling too slowly, rehashing the day's events over and over again. My fulfilment level was at zero. Although I had a number followed by many zeros in my bank account, I didn't have much else. You can only get punched in the face so often before you start to wonder why you always have two black eyes. That was when I started the first of many experiments that would guide my direction over the coming years.

The questions I had been feeding into my mind – 'How can I be more successful?' and 'How can I make more money?' among others – had led to the actions I had taken up to the point, and my life was completely out of balance as a result. I had to own that fact that I wasn't putting the right raw materials into my mind, and I wasn't asking the right questions. Uncomfortably, I had to own the fact that the other areas of my life were suffering because I was focused on the wrong things. All my thoughts were consumed by business, but I wondered why my personal relationships were so poor.

Upon reflection, my habit was analogous to planting apple seeds and then wondering why oranges didn't grow in their place. I had to own the fact that I was focusing on the wrong things. Up until that point, I blamed everybody else for my shortcomings, telling myself that my mental health was poor because that was the price I paid for financial success and that I had no meaningful relationships because people wouldn't work around my schedule. All stories and opinions; none of them were facts. To make any change in your life, you need to take extreme ownership of your life and your shortcomings.

You're overweight? Then you may be consistently consuming too many calories and not burning them off. Cool. Own that. Now you can change it.

You're unhappy? Then you may be consciously or

subconsciously chasing the wrong things or not doing enough things that make you happy. Cool. Own that. Now you can change it.

You're lonely or feel unworthy of love? That's fear manifesting itself in a story that you've told yourself up until now. That's not fact. That's an opinion you hold because of the experiences you've had in the past. Cool. Own that. Now you can change it.

Yes, some people have a genetic predisposition to gain weight easily. Yes, you may have a genuine brain chemistry imbalance that downregulates your brain's happy chemicals. Yes, somebody you loved and trusted may have broken your heart in the past. Certain things in life are genuinely outside of our control, but has any of the self-pity you've been harbouring since helped you? My gut tells me if you're reading this book, it hasn't. It didn't help me either until I made a choice to own my shortcomings.

Just like you can own something or make an excuse for it, you can be a victim or a victor, but you can't be both. The beauty of the situation is that it's your choice. So what are you going to choose?

Remember, if you plant apple seeds, you get apples. If you plant orange seeds, you get oranges. Don't plant apple seeds and expect oranges to grow.

In the next chapter, I present the entire foundation on which my life has been built over the past several years: the four quadrants.

2

Rewire Your Accountability – The Four Quadrants

Accountability structures

The adage 'what gets measured gets managed' is very true, and I've been using accountability structures in my fitness regimens for over seventeen years. I would set a weekly calendar for my meals, my gym workouts and my cardio sessions, and I would cross the tasks off upon completion every day. I did the same for my business. I did calculations for lead generation, developed strategies to hit sales targets and constantly thought about digital marketing to improve conversion rates. From the information I had, I knew that accountability structures worked for me, and random training and nutrition led to random results. The case was the same for business. Therefore, I took that thesis and created an accountability structure for my entire life, leading to the birth of my four-quadrant system.

I spent weeks thinking about how to break up my life. At one point, I created twelve sections with sub-units for each. For all that, I've always subscribed to Einstein's take on simplicity, so I eventually narrowed it down to four quadrants. I knew I couldn't hit a target I couldn't see, so I had to be very clear on what made each of these quadrants successful and what didn't. This thinking resulted in the following personal priorities:

1. Health
2. Wealth
3. Love
4. Fulfilment

In the past two years, I had given about 60% of my time, energy and focus to wealth, 30% to health (physical more than mental) and 5% each to love and fulfilment. Now, I broke up the priorities in my life into four quadrants, with 25% for each quadrant. Although some would and do get more focus depending on the time of the year or current needs, none gets more than 25% overall in terms of my 1–10 rating system.

Every month, I look at the four quadrants on my wall and score them from 1–10.

- How was my health this month? Did I work out four to five times every week (my target)? Did I meditate and relax at least twice every week?
- How was my wealth this month? Did I save and put aside my set target amount over the past thirty days?
- How was my love this month? How much

quality time did I spend on my relevant personal relationships – with my mum, my daughter, my inner circle? Did I get to do my weekly daddy–daughter day with Holly? Did I meet my mum every week?

- How fulfilled did I feel this month? Was the world a better place this month because I was here? Did I help as many people as I could? Did I lose myself in the service of others?

I keep it very simple. If I score an 8 or 9 out of 10 in three quadrants, but a 3 or 4 in another, then the next month I try and bring the low-scoring area back into balance. If my health was a 4 this month because of work commitments, then I prioritise my training sessions and downtime the following month. I started by recording this every day, then every week and now every month. Tell me what you do every day, and I'll tell you where you'll be in a year.

The key to starting the quadrant formula is being honest with yourself. I wasn't very happy when I did it first, as I realised my health was a generous 5 and my wealth a solid 9, but my love and fulfilment were a 2 and 3, respectively.

It doesn't matter where you start; what's important is where you are going. But do not fool yourself or concoct some story that makes you feel okay, such as 'Ah, but I have three kids and don't have the time to work out' or, 'As I have an incredibly stressful job, I just don't have time to meet the right person or see my family or friends. I'll see them during the holidays anyway.' Let's deconstruct these narratives.

First, the above examples are the stories you tell yourself and they are not facts; they're merely opinions. True, maybe you can't prioritise the time to train right now, or you may not have the energy to work out. That's different. Also, you may have a very stressful job, but have you considered the reason your job is so stressful may be that you only think about your job and nothing else? Is it possible that you might feel less stressed if you had someone important in your life with whom you can have a weekend getaway or a weekly family lunch with your loved ones to look forward to? Both are obviously fictitious scenarios, but all I ask of you is that you don't fool yourself with your story. If you're too tired to work out, that's fine, but own that. If you're afraid of dating in case it affects your career negatively, or you're scared of being hurt, that's fine too – but for your own sake, own it. The Nobel Laureate Richard Feynman said it better than I ever can: 'Don't fool yourself and you're the easiest person to fool'.[1]

Leaning into the discomfort of your starting point can be challenging – nobody wants to admit that they're bad at something, particularly if it's something that they value. For example, if you really value your family, but work has been hectic over the last few months, and you haven't spent as much time as you

---

1   R Leighton and R Feynman (1985) *Surely You're Joking Mr Feynman*. New York: Norton and Company.

would have liked with your parents, partner or kids, it can be hard to score the love quadrant at a 3 or a 4. Yet, the key is to be honest with your scoring. Everything you've done is in the past, and you can't change it even if you wanted to, but you can change what you do in the future, and you can change what you do right now.

Also, it's vital to understand that the scoring is completely relative. You're not comparing yourself with anybody else. If you're an advanced athlete who participates in Ironman Triathlons, your criteria to hit a 9 or 10 in the health quadrant is going to be very different from that of someone who's overweight and walks thirty minutes a day.

This leads to my next point – finding what success means to you.

Success in the four quadrants

'You will be a success as soon as you define what success means to you.'
— Jasmine Star

Even if you take nothing else away from the four-quadrant formula apart from finding what success means to you, then you can deem reading the book a worthwhile endeavour. It's easy to get lost in what the external world deems as 'successful'. In the Western world, normally the metrics of success are things like a good job, a considerable amount of money, an attractive partner and a big house. Again, these change from generation to generation and country to country, but that's another reason it's so important to develop your success metrics and define what success looks like to you. If you don't, you will fall into the default definition mentioned above (or some variation of it), climbing the ladder against the wrong wall and wondering why you feel so unfulfilled or unhappy when and if you finally reach the top.

A very simple premise allowed me to devise my success metrics for the four quadrants. First, I compiled a list of all the things that made me happy and the people with whom I loved spending time, and then I actively decided to do more of those things and spend more time with those people. Second, I made a list of all the things that made me unhappy and the people who were negative influences on my life, and I did fewer things that made me unhappy and actively removed or spent less time with the people who brought me down.

If you put Antoine de Saint-Exupéry's principle (which I've paraphrased): 'Perfection comes when there's nothing left to take away, not when there's nothing more to add' into practice every day, you will see how quickly your life begins to change.[2] Your perfect day leads to your perfect week. Your perfect week leads to your perfect month. Your perfect month leads to your perfect year. Perfect years added up lead to an amazing life.

---

2   The original quote is from Antoine de Saint-Exupéry (1942) *Airman's Odyssey*. New York: Reynal & Hitchcock.

Tell me what you do or how you feel every day, and I'll tell you where you'll be or how you'll feel in a year. When you know what success means to you, you can actively put plans in place to either work towards that or live in it right now.

When I started to write up my success metrics, I noticed a really weird thing happening. I was writing them for the future, but I soon realised that most of the things for which I aspired I could give myself right now. I wanted to spend more quality time with my mum, daughter and inner circle. Initially, I was under the impression that I had to 'free up time to have coffee with my mum at least once a week', but as soon as I had written it I thought, 'Wait, I could do that this week!' The same thing happened with my fulfilment aspiration. I wrote, 'I want to find a way to serve thousands of people at once'. A week later, I started my podcast.

I could do nearly all of the things I wanted to do right at the moment. I had been living in my 'I'm too busy' or 'I'll do that when things are less hectic' story for so long. I had forgotten how easy it was to make physical changes in the world when one aligns one's mindset to allow the things you want to happen. Before breaking down my success metrics in each of the four quadrants, I want you to read the following question, pause for 30–60 seconds, close your eyes, ponder the question and just observe the picture that comes to your mind:

'What would I do, have or be right now if I
knew I couldn't fail?'

It doesn't matter what springs to your mind, just don't
get drowned in the 'I can't' or 'It's not realistic' story.
Being realistic is the most-travelled road to mediocrity,
so just cut out all those 'realistic' thoughts rushing into
your mind for the next 30–60 seconds. If you knew
you couldn't fail, and there was no limit, no external
circumstance or experience that could stop it, what
would you do?

Just ask yourself the question:

'What would I do, have or be right now if I
knew I couldn't fail?'

Now wait 30–60 seconds.

Done? Good.

Now, go do that! Or at least never close your mind
off to that possibility again. Your life becomes what
you think about most of the time, and the thoughts to
which you give your energy are going to expand and
manifest. We get so caught up in our story – 'I can't do
this' or 'I can't do that' or 'It isn't realistic' – and we let
that dictate our entire lives. If you peel off the layers of
your story, you'll see that it's grounded and written in
fear – the fear of failure, the fear of success, the fear of
ridicule or social exclusion. In the 'Rewire Fear' chapter,
I will discuss how to reframe fear as a positive emotion
and expand on how the person you want to be is on

the other side of fear; but for now, just question your self-limiting story as that's all it is – a story.

The thoughts you have and the stories you tell yourself manifest themselves in your physical world. If you're not happy with your physical world or any of your four quadrants, then you need to go back to the root. The root of everything in your life to date is an evolved version of the thoughts and actions that preceded it. If you want to change your life, you need to change your actions, but before you do that you need to change your thinking. This applies to all the four quadrants. You may be excelling in three of the four quadrants, but there may be one that's eluding you. Go back to the root on that one and see how you can improve it. When you take new steps, new results will follow them.

The picture you just held in your mind for 30–60 seconds can become real if you let it. Just get out of your own way and 'Don't let your biggest enemy live between your two ears'.

How do my four quadrants look?

Although your four quadrants may look completely different from my own, allow me to give you an example of how mine looks. I update it regularly based on my current goals and priorities, but here is a sample of how it looked in the past. I also provide a step-by-step breakdown of what it takes to hit a 9 or a 10 in a particular quadrant. If you have your own version of the four quadrants or another problem-solving model that you prefer, then feel free to skip straight to the next chapter.

HEALTH

What does health mean to me?
Physical appearance, fitness and overall mental health.

How is it broken up?
1. **Goal 1.** Physical appearance: stay at 10% body fat.
2. **Goal 2.** Fitness: run 50 km every week this month.
3. **Goal 3.** Mental health: feeling fulfilled about and grateful for the things I do have and not focusing on the things I don't have.

What do I need to do to achieve my goals?
Goal 1. Go to the gym four times a week and eat wholegrain foods, some meat or fish, and lots of vegetables and nutrient-dense food.
Goal 2. Run 10 km every evening during the week.
Goal 3. Do 'Digital Detox'* every night before bed.

*Not using any social media, electronics or phones an hour or two before bed to help calm my mind.

What self-created story can hold me back?
Goal 1.
Story: 'I don't have time today.'
Problem: Work or family commitments getting in the way.
Solution: Get up before sunrise and do a gym session before starting work or the family awakes.
Goal 2.
Story: 'It's too cold or wet outside.'
Problem: Weather conditions affecting my run.

Solution: Do the runs on the gym treadmill if needed.

Goal 3.

Story: 'I just need to finish this last piece for work.'

Problem: The desire to keep working late into the night.

Solution: Have a non-negotiable 6pm cut-off time. All computers, social media and phones get powered down at 6pm regardless of how much work is completed.

How do I know I've hit a 9 or 10?

Goal 1. At the end of the month, I've gone to the gym four times every week and eaten high-quality nutrient-dense food 80–90% of the time. I allow myself to eat what I want 10–20% of the time as this strategy helps maintain discipline over the long term.

Goal 2. At the end of the month, I have run a total of 200 km.

Goal 3. At the end of the month, I am sleeping well and feeling energised when I wake up.*

*Note: This is a very personal metric for success. If my mental health is poor, my sleep gets affected, and my energy levels drop. Using that as a gauge tells me how well I did the previous month.

WEALTH

What does wealth mean to me?

Not having to worry about paying my mortgage or bills, and having savings in my bank account in case something bad happens.

How is it broken up?

Goal 1. Earn X amount of money this month to maintain my lifestyle.

Goal 2. Put Y amount away this month to build my savings.

What do I need to do to achieve my goals?

Goal 1. Continue to provide a great service to the people who pay for my products or services.

Goal 2. Pay myself first. Before I pay any bills, as soon as my monthly earnings come into the account, put Y amount into savings, and live off the rest.

What self-created story can hold me back?

Goal 1.

Story: 'I'm too tired today.'

Problem: A poor night of sleep or a hectic schedule is making me less creative or efficient.

Solution: Focus on getting high-quality sleep every night and manage my schedule better by regularly saying 'no' to things that don't help me achieve progress in the four quadrants.

Goal 2.

Story: 'I really want that holiday.'

Problem: Thinking that I can indulge now because I've saved in the past.

Solution: Put money into savings and then create another side pot as a holiday fund. Add to this each month until I have saved enough. It might mean I go to one less dinner that month or spend no money on supplements, but that's fine.

How do I know I've hit a 9 or 10?

Goal 1. At the end of the month, I've served as many people as I could, provided extreme value to them and got paid X amount as a result.

Goal 2. At the end of the month, I have Y amount in my savings account.

LOVE

What does love mean to me?

Spending time with my mum, my daughter and my inner circle of friends and family.

How is it broken up?

Goal 1. Have a weekly daddy–daughter day with my daughter Holly.

Goal 2. Meet my mum for lunch or coffee at least once a week.

Goal 3. Hang out and spend time with at least one person from my inner circle at least once a week.

What do I need to do to achieve my goals?

Goal 1. Take a full day off work. No phone, no work, just me and my daughter doing something that we both enjoy.

Goal 2. Get up early and get my most important tasks finished before 1pm so that I can free up time to meet my mum.

Goal 3. Factor in one half-day off from work and go for food or coffee with someone from my inner circle.

What self-created story can hold me back?

Goal 1, 2, 3.

Story: 'I have a deadline this week. I'll make it up next week.'

Problem: Overcommitting to too many things.

Solution: Say 'no' to everything that doesn't help make progress in any one of the quadrants.

How do I know I've hit a 9 or 10?

Goal 1. At the end of the month, I have a better relationship with my daughter and continue to stay emotionally connected to her as she gets older.

Goal 2. At the end of the month, I've seen my mum nearly every day.

Goal 3. At the end of the month, I feel more emotionally fulfilled after spending time with people who help me grow as a person.

FULFILMENT

What does fulfilment mean to me?

Feeling eager to jump out of bed every morning, working a job I love and connecting with amazing people.

How is it broken up?

Goal 1. Write four chapters of the new book (the one you're currently reading).

Goal 2. Create effective podcasts with guests who inspire or educate my audience and me.

What do I need to do to achieve my goals?

Goal 1. Prioritise 'writing time' every morning for the next month.

Goal 2. Keep an eye out for inspiring personalities with whom I can connect for my podcast.

What self-created story can hold me back?

Goal 1.

Story: 'I'll write that chapter another day. I can't get in the zone today.'

Problem: Being lazy because writing doesn't come as easily to me as speaking.

Solution: Sit down and write regardless of how I feel. Even if the work is below par, sit down every single morning and just write. Sometimes, one has to work one's way into the zone.

Goal 2.
Story: 'That person isn't right for my show.'
Problem: Not doing enough research on potential guests.
Solution: Spend at least sixty minutes researching potential guests and find the best fits for the show.

How do I know I've hit a 9 or 10?
Goal 1. At the end of the month, I've completed four new chapters of the book.
Goal 2. At the end of the month, I've inspired and educated others and myself with the podcast guests with whom I've connected.

Again, the aspects mentioned above are just examples, and your priorities, goals and strategies may be completely different. It's worth noting that they can change regularly based on the time of year or your current priorities. If I'm working on a book with an imminent deadline or have a lot of back-to-back talks in a single month, I may scale back my goals in another quadrant. For example, when writing this book, I completely cut out Goal 2 from the health quadrant. I didn't have any races coming up, so I didn't need to set aside an hour a day for running. Instead, I spent the time writing or editing a section of this book. Therefore, doing this evaluation every month is important as one's priorities change regularly.

After a while, you may not even need to write it out every single month. I don't anymore, but it helps to do it in the beginning to get you started. I did it every single month for the first six months, and now it's automatic and has become just a habit.

Here's a blank list you can fill out.

HEALTH
What does health mean to me?

How is it broken up?
Goal 1. ....
Goal 2. ....
Goal 3. ....

What do I need to do to achieve my goals?
Goal 1. ....
Goal 2. ....
Goal 3. ....

What self-created story can hold me back?
Goal 1: ....
Story: ....
Problem: ....
Solution: ....
Goal 2: ....
Story: ....
Problem: ....
Solution: ....
Goal 3: ....
Story: ....
Problem: ....
Solution: ....

How do I know I've hit a 9 or 10?
Goal 1. ....
Goal 2. ....
Goal 3. ....

WEALTH

What does wealth mean to me?

How is it broken up?
Goal 1. ....
Goal 2. ....
Goal 3. ....

What do I need to do to achieve my goals?
Goal 1. ....
Goal 2. ....
Goal 3. ....

What self-created story can hold me back?
Goal 1. ....
Story: ....
Problem: ....
Solution: ....
Goal 2. ....
Story: ....
Problem: ....
Solution: ....
Goal 3. ....
Story: ....
Problem: ....
Solution: ....

How do I know I've hit a 9 or 10?
Goal 1...
Goal 2...
Goal 3...

LOVE

What does love mean to me?

How is it broken up?
Goal 1...
Goal 2...
Goal 3...

What do I need to do to achieve my goals?
Goal 1...
Goal 2...
Goal 3...

What self-created story can hold me back?
Goal 1...
Story:..
Problem:..
Solution:...
Goal 2...
Story:..
Problem:..
Solution:...
Goal 3...
Story:..
Problem:..
Solution:...

How do I know I've hit a 9 or 10?
Goal 1...
Goal 2...
Goal 3...

FULFILMENT
What does fulfilment mean to me?

How is it broken up?
Goal 1...
Goal 2...
Goal 3...

What do I need to do to hit my goals?
Goal 1...
Goal 2...
Goal 3...

What self-created story can hold me back?
Goal 1...
Story:..
Problem:..
Solution:..
Goal 2...
Story:..
Problem:..
Solution:..
Goal 3...
Story:..
Problem:..
Solution:..

How do I know I've hit a 9 or 10?

Goal 1. ....

Goal 2. ....

Goal 3. ....

3

Rewire Your Confidence

Dealing with self-doubt

As mentioned earlier, confidence comes from saying you're going to do something and then actually going and doing it. However, confidence and self-doubt are on opposite sides of the pendulum. The more self-doubt you have, the less confident you tend to be, and the more confidence you have, the less self-doubt you tend to have.

Building legs on that confidence table doesn't happen overnight. One doesn't wake up one fine morning and go from being insecure and full of self-doubt to brimming with confidence and unwavering belief; it just doesn't work like that. One of the reasons I struggled so much with self-doubt in the early part of my life was my inability to delay gratification. I wanted everything now! I wanted the perfect body now. I wanted more money now. I wanted to have all the external things I thought would make me successful now. Such an impatient attitude led me to make stupid decisions in the hopes of forcing things to happen quickly. Financially, I went broke three times before I turned twenty-five. I overused recreational fat burners to try and get leaner so that I would feel more confident. I imposed huge caloric restrictions (ie, eating very little food) on myself to look good in a nightclub on a Saturday night. All of these were the plasters on my self-doubt because I was too mentally weak to accept the truth: Nothing happens overnight.

I frequently mention habits in this book because one is what one repeatedly does. If you constantly look for shortcuts instead of doing the work, then don't complain if it all blows up in your face. The tendencies to take shortcuts and look for quick fixes are due to the victim mentality, and I was the worst kind of victim. I would first look for quick fixes and, when they inevitably failed, I blamed everybody else for them not working out. I never owned the fact that I made the decision in the first place.

It's human nature to lean towards taking responsibility for the positive things in our lives and distance ourselves from the negative things that happen to us. We tell ourselves that we have good jobs because we studied and worked hard for them. We're in good shape because we eat well and work out regularly. We are in loving relationships because we're loyal, trustworthy and faithful. Although all these things may be true, you may not be looking at the full picture if you position the bad things as being outside of your control.

When bad things happen, we tend to blame somebody or something else. Yes, you may have a lot going for you, but you tell yourself that there are no good men or women out there, and that's why you're single. You may tell yourself you're miserable in your job because your boss doesn't recognise your talents. I've seen this pattern in so many people's lives, and I did exactly the same thing! I gave myself credit for being in great physical shape, but I blamed the economy for not being able to set up my own business. Once the business worked out, I blamed a lack of time for not having any meaningful relationships. All stories, all opinions, none of them true, but I felt good blaming something or somebody other than myself.

If you don't take ownership of the bad things in your life, you don't deserve to take responsibility for the good things in your life. You can't have it both ways. Either none of them are due to your efforts and all of them are due to 'luck', or all of them are because of you and the decisions you made, the good and the bad.

Two major points of focus helped in dealing with my self-doubt. The first was taking responsibility for everything that happened to me. True, you can't help if your partner cheated on you or if you were bullied as a kid or even if a work colleague did you a bad turn once, but you can control the story you wrap around it. You can choose to see the bitter experience as a lesson and use the feedback from it to make better decisions in the future. Your partner cheated on you, but now you know what signs to look for in your next relationship. Somebody beat the crap out of you when you were a kid, but now you can use that fire to grow mentally and physically stronger. A work colleague did you a bad turn, but now you know the kind of person that you can or can't trust going forward. All failures provide feedback if you choose to look for it.

The second point of focus came from my love of studying history. As a former teacher, history was one of my favourite topics to teach, and although I don't work in the traditional education system anymore, I still read history all the time. The more history I read, the more I realised that history doesn't necessarily repeat itself, but it sure as hell rhymes.[1]

The story of the artist Michelangelo who painted the Sistine Chapel is one that always serves me when dealing with self-doubt. Michelangelo was an Italian Renaissance sculptor, painter, architect, and poet. He is best known for the famed sculpture *David* and the ceiling of the Sistine Chapel in Vatican City. Michelangelo was and still is known as one of the greatest artists to have ever lived. Although better known for his work as a sculptor, he was asked by Pope Julius II to paint the frescoes on the ceiling of the Sistine Chapel. Hesitant at first, he eventually agreed.

His hesitancy largely stemmed from the fact that murals such as the one in the Sistine Chapel are to be completed while the plaster is still wet. In other words, he had to get the paintings right on the first attempt

---

[1] This quip is often attributed to Mark Twain, although there's no evidence he actually made it.

as there was no option to redo it, leaving no room for mistakes. While painting, Michelangelo was plagued with self-doubt. Being an artist who specialised in sculpting, he regularly questioned his ability in other art forms.

The story goes that one night, Michelangelo, being completely exhausted, climbed down the scaffolding and lay down to rest. After eating a lonely supper, he wrote a sonnet to his aching body, mumbling to himself, 'I am no painter'.[2] He felt so challenged and deterred by his own feeling of self-doubt that he believed he was a terrible painter.

Every time I question my ability as a writer, speaker or coach, I remember Michelangelo's words, and it helps me deal with my own self-doubt. It always serves me to know that one of the greatest painters of all time questioned his painting ability.

Reading that story for the first time made me realise that everyone has self-doubt, even the greats. Learning to ignore the voice in your head saying that you can't do it is crucial to getting your ladder up against the right wall. Understanding that self-doubt doesn't go away has made the biggest difference to me over the past several years. We all have self-doubt in certain areas of life, but the key is to acknowledge the self-doubt, feel the fear and do it anyway.

---

2   This is from Michelangelo to Giovanni Da Pistoia in G Mazur (2005) *Zeppo's First Wife: New and selected poems.* Chicago: University of Chicago Press.

One of my tools to stay on course when self-doubt creeps in is using the acronym WIN – What's Important Now.

It may take years to master yourself and your inner thoughts, but when you focus on What's Important Now (WIN) even the biggest goals can be broken down into the smallest tasks. If you're trying to lose 100 lbs of weight, don't focus on the end goal of 100 lbs; instead, focus on first losing 1 lb, then 2 lbs, then 3 lbs. If you want to run a marathon, don't focus on the end goal of 26.2 miles; rather, focus on running 1 mile, then 2 miles, and so on. By doing a task step by step, we get ahead figuratively and literally.

Once you apply the philosophy that nothing happens overnight and the struggle makes the victory even sweeter, then success becomes almost inevitable. We have the ability to make conscious decisions to change our attitudes, our skill sets and our lives. Again, it just comes down to learning to control negative self-talk and changing the way you see things.

Here is another exercise that can be incredibly effective but may be uncomfortable to do – asking others what weaknesses they see in you. Remember to ask them to be brutally honest. From personal experience, this exercise isn't easy, but it can be very helpful in making us see our blind spots (ie, the characteristics that we fail to see in ourselves but that are so obvious to others). The key is to do it with the people you trust who want to see you improve. I do this exercise with the people in my inner circle regularly.

In the beginning, the feedback you get can be difficult to take. I remember being told the first time I asked that I was self-absorbed and too obsessed with being successful and that I failed to prioritise the people closest to me, and it hurt a lot. And it hurt because it was true. Still, the honest feedback helped me realise that I put myself above others when it came to making decisions, and my drive was focused on the accumulation of things: cars, clothes, status – basically all the things I thought would make me feel superior to others.

I like to think of such conversations as one's first workout in the gym or the first time one does any new physical exercise. The first workout is always painful, leaving us sore for a few days. Afterwards, as we become more adapted to the training, we become stronger. Like the gym makes us physically stronger, having difficult conversations makes us mentally and emotionally stronger. Therefore, lean into the discomfort of uncomfortable conversations and see how quickly your life begins to change for the better. As the quote often attributed to Vincent Van Gogh says, 'The comfort zone is a beautiful place, but nothing ever grows there'. I'll go one step further and say the discomfort zone is a beautiful place because everything grows there!

Asking for criticism may seem counterintuitive to working on your self-doubt, but facing these insecurities makes you mentally tougher. When you own your weaknesses, wear them as badges of honour and begin to improve upon them, your self-confidence will skyrocket, eliminating all your self-doubt.

Remember, in the moment of painting the Sistine Chapel, even Michelangelo believed himself to be a worthless painter. Reviewing who he became and his overall accomplishments, we now know him to be one of the best painters in all of history. Therefore, don't let your self-doubt determine your self-worth.

If getting your ladder up against the right wall is the first step, and getting over your self-doubt and building confidence are the second and third steps in rewiring your mindset, then the next obstacle you need to tackle is caring too much about what other people think about you. Learning to inoculate yourself from the opinion of others, especially those whose opinions don't really matter, can free you to do all the things that make you happy.

No-complaining zone

I'm reaching out to all the people who are living like I was, complaining about their lives, feeling like victims, believing life is something that happened to them and not for them. If you're not happy with where you are, who you are or what you have, you can move and change; you are not a tree!

Complaining about your situation is just a discreet way of playing the victim. True, you are not repeating 'woe is me' – the traditional mindset we associate with victims – but complaining is much more dangerous as it hides the truth of what you are really doing.

Complaining is the mask you wear when you want to be a victim but can't or don't want to admit it.

Tell me what you do every day, and I'll tell you where you'll be in a year, five years or ten years. When I see people constantly complaining about their situation – their job, their relationship, their health, body or fitness level – I know 95% of them are going to be in the same place in five or ten years, complaining about something else – or, worse, the same thing. Nothing changes until you start making new decisions. If you're that person, you can change, and I implore you to do so.

Who you have been up until now isn't who you are becoming. If you're reading this book and you're what I call a 'cloaked complainer' – your cloak or mask covers your victim mentality – then consciously decide to make yourself one of the 5% who decide to own it, control it and change it.

Also, don't beat yourself up if that's how you've been up until now. I was one of that 95% and was the king of excuses and a cloaked complainer for years, so you're in good company. But when I became aware of it, I decided to change it. That's it.

The above discussion brings me to my next point: Should you ever complain? Does it have any benefits?

The truth is that if you can go through the rest of your life without complaining, you will probably be much better off. I had to start small. I undertook a thirty-day no-complaining challenge to see how badly ingrained my tendency to complain was.

The challenge is exactly as it sounds – no complaining for thirty days. I told all my closest friends I was doing it and gave them permission to call me out if I faltered. Also, if I found myself complaining mid-sentence, I would pause and say out loud, 'No complaining for thirty days'.

I'm not going to lie to you; seeing the challenge through was incredibly difficult! The first time I tried the challenge, I was already pretty good at owning everything I did, and I wouldn't have classified myself as a 'complainer'. Yet, when I started the challenge I realised I had a few default complaints that I was unaware of – running late for meetings because of traffic or giving out about a situation because of the weather. I didn't even realise I had been doing it until that point. After three days, I set 'no-complaining zone' as the screensaver on my phone, which helped considerably. As my phone was nearly always within my arms' reach, every time I unlocked the screen it served as a subtle visual reminder of my task for the day.

At the end of thirty days, I had significantly reduced my 'mini complaints' and was able to stop myself mid-sentence and rewire my mindset about nearly any given situation. If it was raining outside, I would catch myself mid-sentence and remind myself, 'Yes, it's raining, but a blind man would love to see it all the same', or if I heard somebody else complain about the weather to me, I would reply, 'The weather may be bad, but the day is awesome'. It's worth noting that the first time you respond like that, it tends to be such a major pattern interruption that most people don't know how to respond and just look at you blankly for a while. It's fun to experiment with this challenge for the reactions alone!

You may read this and wonder how this one little change of not complaining about the weather helped my life in any way, shape or form. My reply: 'Tell me how you do the small things, and I'll tell you how you'll handle the big things'. I am confident that if you train yourself not to complain about the weather or small things, you'll notice how you stop complaining about all the big things too – your boss, your husband or wife, your work colleagues, among others. How you do anything is how you do everything. Complaining is for victims. Being a complainer is probably the subtlest version of being a victim, as the complaints are hidden beyond a cloak of discontent or subconscious default mechanisms hardwired over the years.

Also, we associate a victim with someone who is passive, not doing anything or being quiet and timid. On the contrary, the active form of complaining is as much, if not more, the mindset of a victim than that of a quiet, timid person who figuratively curls up in the corner afraid of the world. The danger is that you won't recognise and see such tendencies as they're not what you generally associate with 'being a victim'. Don't be fooled!

Remember that how you handle the small things

is how you will handle the big things. Start with the thirty-day no-complaining challenge or even a three-day or three-hour no-complaining challenge and take ownership of your problems. You can't change what you don't own.

4

Rewire Seeking Approval – How to Stop Caring About What People Think of You

Trigger words to set you off

'To avoid criticism, say nothing, do nothing, be nothing.'
— Elbert Hubbard

When insulted, people typically become angry. This is a character flaw I have spent years trying to iron out in myself as it switches my mind from a rational state where I am able to make clear decisions about the best thing to do in any given situation to an emotional state where my anger or annoyance takes control. Generally, at this point, my mind would shut off to any new information, and I would automatically go into defence mode. If someone questioned my physical training method or nutritional protocol preference or character, I would either respond irrationally and then be left to clean up the pieces and apologise after I had calmed down or let the insult fester and build inside me, never realising that being angry or annoyed at someone else was like drinking poison myself and expecting the other person to die.

I remember one such incident with my sister, who is one of the closest people to me and part of my inner circle. She and I had a bitter argument that resulted in her labelling me as 'boring'.

I describe myself as a social introvert. I love people and tremendously enjoy hearing their stories and talking to them about their dreams and ambitions, but my figurative battery recharges when I am left alone. Although I have addressed audiences of thousands of people, I dislike being in the middle of big crowds even to this day and have to actively 'feel the fear and do it anyway'. If it were up to me, I would always opt for a small gathering of five to ten people over a party of a hundred.

On this one occasion, my sister and I were due to attend a party of about a hundred friends and family members. I thought about going and agreed to do so, only to back out at the last minute, owing to my conflict avoidance tendencies and my inability to say 'no'. My behaviour got my sister annoyed, so she called me 'boring'. This is what I call a 'trigger' word. A trigger word is any word that fills you with anger or discomfort as soon as it's uttered, often due to an emotional, physical or mental trauma from childhood or adolescence.

Now I know that 'boring' is a trigger word for me.

Although being called that doesn't override my rational mind like it once did, at the time it set me off like a loose cannon. I didn't speak to my sister for weeks, all over my inability to deal with what I perceived to be a challenge to my character or a direct insult. Ten years later, I can laugh about my reaction as I now know she used it as a throwaway comment, not meaning to offend me or set me off. She could not have known that it was a trigger word for me. Even I didn't know it at the time. That's why self-awareness and the ability to identify the things, people or words that make you feel angry or annoyed are so critical in having a happier life. Once you identify the problem, you can decide to own it, and from there you can change it if you choose to.

To give you a bit of a background as to why the particular word set me off, I need to take you back a few years. I was bullied quite badly as a teenager. I suffered from a skin condition that caused terrible acne and countless spots, which scarred my face, neck and body. The other kids at school called me 'crater face' and 'spot boy' for the first half of my high school years. Moreover, although I played sports, I was quite small until I turned about sixteen. I channelled my focus towards sports as it was my form of escapism, and it was and still is my mechanism to enter the 'flow' state where I completely lose track of time. Therefore, I never drank alcohol or partied too hard as a teenager. I more than made up for the abstinence during my university years, but in my teenage years, it came at a social cost. Along with the names pertaining to my dermatological issues, 'boring' was also regularly used to taunt and bully me. Soon, the words 'spot boy' and 'boring' become synonymous in my mind. My skin cleared up before I left for university, so I never heard the insult 'spot boy' ever again. Still, the emotional turmoil and mild depression I felt at the time comes alive a little bit every time someone calls me 'boring' since the word is so tightly linked with the feelings from the time. This anecdote shows you the power of words and how they can be hardwired in our limbic system, serving as just another example of how powerful your self-talk is and the mental thought seeds you plant.

Not until I was in my early twenties did I realise that 'boring' was a trigger word capable of sending me from a rational state to an emotional one in the blink of an eye. We all have such trigger words, and some are significantly worse and more obvious than others. For example, once I was at a football game with one of my closest friends from London, who is of Jamaican heritage, and a group of inebriated teenagers started hurling abuse – including the 'N-word' – at my friend. To my surprise, he maintained his composure, exhibiting a remarkable ability to contain himself. He just turned to me and said, 'That word used to set me off once upon a time but not anymore. I've taken ownership of the word so that nobody can hurt me with it. Besides, the kids probably don't even know the cultural history around it.' His reaction is something I still greatly admire to this day and serves as personal inspiration to me when dealing with any negative comments.

Please note that I'm not comparing trigger words like 'boring' to the 'N-word'. I understand they can't be further apart in terms of meanings and connotations. One is used to hurt and offend people on the basis of race, which can never be condoned. The other just refers to a personality trait. The reason I bring it up is to illustrate how some trigger words are really obvious; they offend because of the historical and cultural connotations around them. However, other words are not so obvious, and they serve as triggers due to emotional events or traumas attached to them for individuals.

I like to think of my rational and emotional sides as the two ends of a spectrum, with rational at 1 and emotional at 10 on the scale:

Rational   Emotional

1   2   3   4   5   6   7   8   9   10

I like to stay at a 1 or 2 all day unless I'm supporting my favourite team at a sporting event or watching a movie, as that's structured emotional time where I let inhibitions go and just enjoy the experience. On the contrary, when I'm making business or life decisions, the more rational I am the better my decisions tend to be.

The reason I am sharing this spectrum with you is that it can be very useful in helping identify your 'trigger' words. Ask yourself what words move you from a 1 or 2 to a 9 or a 10 as soon as they are uttered? 'Fat', 'ugly', 'small', 'skinny', 'stupid', 'selfish' and 'needy' are some recognisable examples, but yours may be as subtle as 'boring', 'shy', 'loud' or 'brash'.

Keep note of the words that affect you. As someone whose life has changed profoundly and whose relationships have improved dramatically by just identifying this one factor, I wanted to share it in the book.

Removing the sting of insults

The writings of Seneca and other stoic philosophers helped me immensely in developing the strategies to deal with my issues. As anger is a negative emotion that can upset one's tranquillity, the Stoics thought it worthwhile to develop the strategies to prevent insults from angering us – strategies for removing the sting of insults.

One of their sting-elimination strategies is to pause, when insulted, to consider whether the insulting statement is true. If it is, there is little reason to be upset. For example, suppose someone mocks you for being bald when you are, in fact, bald. In such a case, Seneca asks, 'Why is it an insult to be told what is self-evident?'[1]

If I could go back to the difficult situation my fourteen-year-old self faced, I would tell myself the same: 'Yes, you have terrible acne but it will probably go away when you're older, and yes, people are saying nasty things to you, but that's their way of dealing with their insecurities. It's a reflection of them, not of you.'

I wish this were only the case for adolescents or

---

1   W B Irvine (2008) *A Guide to the Good Life: The ancient art of stoic joy.* Oxford: Oxford University Press.

teenagers, but the same problem follows us throughout our adult lives. We get offended when people call us names even if there's some truth in it. If someone calls you fat, and you are in fact three stone over your ideal weight, then own it and try to change it. If someone tells you that you're not smart or intelligent in the traditional sense, own it and make efforts to change it by improving your intellectual abilities if you so choose. Even if you don't go into how other people project their insecurities onto you, you can turn your focus inward and control your reaction entirely. Let them call you names or tell you that you can't do something – that's on them, not you. I do want you to ask one question, though: Why did it affect you in the first place?

The purple polar bear

Picture yourself walking down a street on a sunny morning. The birds are chirping, and you're feeling pretty good about how your life is going at the moment. You're just back from a holiday and have a lovely new tan that's making you feel pretty confident. Suddenly, you feel your phone vibrating in your pocket. It's the notification for a comment on one of your recent holiday pictures: 'I see somebody enjoyed themselves. Don't worry; I'm sure that holiday weight will fall right off.' Instantly you've gone from being in a pretty good mood, admiring the singing birds, to being in a disturbed mood. The inner dialogue, 'Oh God, they're right. I have put on so much weight', or 'I should take down the picture', or the defensive 'F*ck that person', will resound in your mind.

Some variation of this story has happened to nearly everyone. Sometimes it's at a party or social gathering, sometimes it's while you're out on the street, but the situation is the same. One moment you're feeling pretty good, and suddenly an external comment or stimulus, real or virtual, alters your mood. The nature of the insult may change – someone may call you stupid or ugly or make passive-aggressive comments like 'You're lucky that you're good-looking' or 'Don't quit your day job', but the principle is the same. You feel fine one moment, but your emotions shift the next. You go from happy and content to frustrated, upset, insecure or angry. If you're like most people, such comments will eat away at you for hours. You will probably jump back and forth between defending yourself and internally attacking the person who made the comment to a downward spiral of agreeing with them and contemplating your worth altogether. Now I have two questions for you: Why does the comment affect you, and why does it make you insecure, frustrated, upset or angry?

Before delving into the reason for your reaction, let's picture the exact scenario again but with one simple variation. One fine morning, you're walking down a street, feeling happy about life and your new tan. Feeling a vibration in your pocket, you take out your phone and click the notification for a comment. The comment reads, 'You're a purple polar bear'. Now, what's your reaction? If you're like most people, your reaction will be 'WTF? That person is crazy! What are they even talking about?' and you will soon forget about it. Now, here's an interesting question: Why didn't the comment make you feel frustrated, angry, insecure or upset? Why didn't the comment affect you?

This was and continues to be one of the most difficult questions I ask myself. 'Purple polar bear' is just a random collection of words. It could just as easily be 'green desert penguin'. We don't have any emotional attachment to either; neither is a reflection of us, and the words are meaningless. They not a reflection of us, but they also don't contain any of our insecurities. It's only when our insecurities are put out there for the world to see, on social media, at a family gathering or while walking down the street, that we feel that strong emotional connection to what has been said.

In my first book, *The Fitness Mindset*, I discussed how we tend to get attached to the words other people throw at us and hold onto them like our first-born child, never realising that they're just opinions. The inoculation against such tendencies is realising that opinions change over time when more information is given and separating facts from opinions. However, when comments affect you, it's normally due to one of the two following reasons:

1. The comment triggered an insecurity of yours
2. The person is correct in what they're saying, and they've identified a personality trait you're not happy to own yet

When competing as a bodybuilder and professional fitness model, I held what I call 'junk values' – values that are selfish and don't really improve the lives of others in any meaningful way. In the 'Rewire Self-sabotage' chapter, I speak about the 'value ladder' and the importance of understanding what's valuable to you, but back in 2014, at the height of my competitive fitness career, most of my values were junk.

The way I looked, in particular, was at the top of my value ladder. I spent most of my time figuring out how I could get leaner, bigger and more defined, and my actions mapped onto my goals. I trained several hours a day, ate meals every three hours and put other parts of my life on hold. As I mention throughout this book, what you focus on is what will expand. I focused on these goals, and they are what expanded. But, as the way I physically looked was so important to me, anyone who challenged that was normally met with extreme defensiveness or an all-out attack from my side.

I remember an incident from 2014 when I was in the middle of a training session about four weeks out from a bodybuilding show. I had been dieting hard for about twelve weeks at that point and felt I looked pretty good. My body fat was low, I looked lean and I was feeling pretty confident that my hard work was paying off. As I was changing after my workout, one of the other gym members looked at me and said, 'Didn't your legs used to be a lot bigger?' That was it, nothing too sinister, just a passing throwaway comment. He meant nothing by it and was merely making an observation. Yet, at the time, so much of my self-esteem was wrapped up in the way I looked that I spent the next five minutes looking at my legs in the mirror. Then, my negative self-talk kicked in, and the imposter syndrome started to circle my mind: 'He's right! Your legs are too small. What are you thinking even doing another show? You're not good enough. You're not big enough' and on and on. Eventually, those thoughts turned me into the man with a hammer (as the saying goes: to the man with a hammer, the whole world looks like a nail), and I went on an attack. My attitude was 'F*ck that guy! What does he know?'

It's funny because you may never compete in a bodybuilding show or even care about your physical appearance, and yet you've probably lived through a similar experience. If being smart, funny or witty is of value to you, as soon as someone questions your intelligence, humour or quickness of reply, you'll feel the same way I did.

At that point of time, instead of getting to the source of why a comment affected me (like I do now), I would bury my head in the sand and try to ignore it. The strategy was okay for the short term, but inevitably the same thing would happen with another body part.

If you put the same insecure person into a new body, a new car or new clothes, they're still going to be insecure. Now they just have a better body, a nicer car or cooler clothes. The secret is to question why those comments affected you in the first place. Going back to the anecdote, in my head, being big, lean and fit meant that I would do well at shows. Doing well at shows meant I would get more work as a fitness model. Getting more work as a fitness model would show people how successful I was. Showing people how successful I was would make people respect me. People respecting me would make me feel worthy. Peeling off the layers of my action, as I talked about in the 'Rewire Your Accountability' chapter, I realised I didn't have a bigger-legs issue but a self-worth issue.

The comment affected me only because I had an emotional attachment to what the comment addressed. If the guy in the dressing room had called me 'a purple polar bear', it would have washed straight over me, but his words affected me for a reason. The next time somebody calls you something that affects you, don't ignore it and bury your head in the sand. Ponder why it hit you, and you may find a golden message hidden in it. Some of the most significant milestones in my personal growth have come from leaning into that uncomfortable reality. I hated admitting I had a self-worth issue as it made me feel weak and helpless. The irony was that all great strength comes from weakness and admitting a weakness is the opposite of helplessness. Owning it allowed me to control it and controlling it allowed me to change it.

Fast forward several years, and I don't have any emotional attachment to the way I look anymore. If somebody calls me too big, too small, too lean or too fat, it all washes over me like somebody calling me a purple polar bear.

This only happened because when we ask ourselves why something affects us, we can get to the root of the problem. When we get to the root, which was self-worth in my case, then we can own that weakness and change it. The next time someone tells you something that affects you, don't run from it and don't bury your head in the sand. Ask yourself, 'Why did that affect me?' Once you have that information, you can decide what you want to do with it. Then, I always use a follow-up question when something affects me: 'Are they right in what they're saying?'

Are they right?

Another sting-elimination strategy suggested by Epictetus, another favourite stoic of mine, is to pause to consider how well informed the insulters are.[2] They may be saying something bad about you not because they want to hurt your feelings but because they sincerely believe what they are saying, or they may simply be reporting how things seem to them. Rather than getting angry with them for their honesty, you should calmly set them straight. When I get annoyed with somebody just because they hold what I feel is a skewed or narrow opinion of me, I repeat the following mantra: 'They are doing the best they can with the information they currently have'.

---

2   A Long (2002) *Epictetus: A stoic and socratic guide to life*. Oxford: Clarendon Press.

As someone who puts his thoughts, opinions and perspectives out there for the entire world to see, agree with or criticise, sometimes the negative comments aimed at my direction are true from the commenter's particular perspective. In fact, I love constructive criticism; it's a contextual reframe strategy for helping me to improve in my craft or art but something I've had to work on as my natural or 'default' mode doesn't handle criticism very well.

When I started my business, I believed in the line: 'The only taste of success some people get is when they take a bite out of you', and to some extent that is true. Small people will always try to bring you down to their level; though, this isn't necessarily the most supportive belief system to have. Closing my mind off to criticism made it nearly impossible for me to improve. It's too easy to put all the criticism into the same box and then close it. You strike gold when you are able to separate the negative criticism from the constructive criticism.

I remember receiving some great constructive criticism about the interviewing techniques I used in my podcasts, for which I have interviewed some of the world's top health professionals, sports stars and various experts and deconstructed what made them so successful. Having grown up on a farm in the West of Ireland, I have a pretty bad habit of swearing in my default speech, which is common among farmers (though normally attributed to sailors). It's a trait I have ironed out over the years. I have done full keynote speeches and long-form interviews without uttering a single swear word, but if you give me two or three beers, my language goes straight back to the default mode.

My tendency to swear came up in an interview I did once. I was speaking with Damian Browne, a former professional rugby player who had just finished rowing solo across the Atlantic Ocean. Damian is a soft-spoken, gentle giant. He is about 270 lbs, 6'7 and doesn't swear all that often. I, on the other hand, have very high energy, and although I've worked on calming down over the years when the occasion warrants it, it's not something that comes to me very naturally. During the interview, I was my normal high-energy self, and Damian was his regular soft-spoken, calm self. The interview went great, and I left it at that. However, a week after the podcast went live, I received an email from a listener explaining how he loved my podcast and the interview with Damian, but he found the tonality differences very off-putting. He added that I swore more than my guest, and it might be worth considering trying to match my guests' tone as to ensure a better interview flow. He also suggested that I shouldn't swear if the guest doesn't, as it makes me seem 'brash' in comparison. I listened to the interview again and realised he had made some very good points. Since then, I've always tried to match the tone and flow of the guest with whom I'm speaking, and as a result, I feel I now have a much better and more balanced interview style.

Had those comments come three years prior, my

default reaction would have been to shut them out, label the email sender a 'hater' and then just carry on with what I was doing, missing the opportunity to learn and improve.

Every criticism is a chance to get better. If you don't agree with the words aimed at your direction, then talk directly to your critic and see why they see it so from that perspective. Again, use your energy wisely. There's a saying in business circles that 'you can't sell the unsellable' – if somebody isn't willing to meet you halfway or they're not open to having more information or dialogue to potentially change their opinion of you or your ideas, then move on.

I think of changing the minds of unreceptive people like trying to teach a pig how to fly. Only two things really happen when you try to teach a pig to fly: 1) The pig doesn't learn how to fly, and 2) you just annoy the pig. If someone's mind is closed off to changing their opinion of you or what you do, then move on; don't waste your energy, and don't try to sell the unsellable. Oink, oink!

Why are you taking advice from someone you wouldn't trade places with?

Another effective sting-elimination strategy is to consider the source of an insult. If you respect the critics and value their opinions, then their critical remarks shouldn't upset you. For example, several years ago I hired business mentors to support me in taking my fitness business to the next level. In this case, I was paying them to criticise me. It would be utterly foolish, under those circumstances, for me to respond to their criticism with hurt feelings. On the contrary, as I was serious about learning how to improve my business and serve more people on a grander scale and had previously reframed criticism as a positive thing, I regularly thanked them for unsympathetic feedback.

Suppose, though, that you don't respect your critics. In that case, why are you even listening to them in the first place? My general rule is: if I won't switch places with my critics, then I shouldn't be taking advice from them.

Of course, there are exceptions to the rule. A competent personal trainer might be currently out of shape due to an injury; an amazing prospective partner may be currently out of a relationship due to circumstance or refusing to settle below their standards; a business guru may have made one bad unhedged financial decision that led to short-term bankruptcy. But they all may still have the wisdom and experience to support you on your journey. Sometimes, imagining yourself in these scenarios is even better than imagining switching places with someone more 'successful' as you can learn from their mistakes as well. The key is to be aware of who you are listening to or taking advice from.

When I talk about the people you won't trade places with, I'm referring to your friends and family who have an opinion on everything. Your friend 'Jane', who is three stone overweight and has been 'yo-yo' dieting for four years, mocks you for going to the gym four days a week, eating several small meals a day and getting into a mild calorie deficit when, according to her, you can just take a bar or shake for three months and lose all the weight faster. In such a case, let Jane do her thing, but don't let her views influence your decisions. She is expressing an opinion, not stating a fact. Her opinion is that you should go on a juice or bar diet and lose weight quickly (albeit to rebound back after a month of eating normal food again), but her advice hasn't even helped her, so why would it help you? Jane may be your best friend and an amazing person; she may even be the most emotionally intelligent person you know and gives great relationship or life advice, but she is not the ideal person to take dietary advice from. It may sound obvious, but we all take unhelpful advice to heart. I've done it myself.

For example, I struggled with romantic relationships for years, during most of my early and mid-twenties. Who do you think I took advice from when trying to improve that area of my life? Surely, people whose relationships have stood the test of time or friends with whom I would have switched places? Unfortunately not. In fact, I did quite the opposite. I went looking for advice from my other single friends who were no better or worse off than I was. I don't think I need to elaborate on how stupid my strategy was or is, but I will sometimes still indulge in it anyway.

It's almost instinctive to ask your friends, family members or peers for their opinions on a problem or situation. This innate tendency to seek everybody's 'two cents' is another reason why it's so important to understand that you are the average of the five people with whom you spend the most time. When seeking advice on your diet, a job opportunity or your love life from another person, ask yourself the simple question, 'Would I switch places with this person?' If the answer is no, then you have to consider how much weight you give to their opinion.

Let me explain how such tendencies manifested in my life. I would meet a new woman whom I liked, invite her to meet my friends and ask what they thought of her, but time and time again they would find some fault with her, and I would break it off. I learned two very valuable lessons from these experiences. One is obviously not to seek advice from the people with whom I wouldn't switch places, and the second is never to let other people's opinions cloud my judgement.

For me, it was and still is important that my friends like my girlfriend, partner or wife, but their opinions can't carry so much weight that they cloud my judgement of someone else. The key to making good decisions is to weigh all the valuable information in front of you, weigh the upsides, weigh the downsides, ask yourself whether you can handle the downsides and then make the decision yourself. This is the strategy I followed when I left my teaching job to start my personal training business, and it's still the strategy I use today when making everyday decisions.

Nevertheless, it took me years to understand this

as I kept repeating the same mistakes over and over. It wasn't until I switched strategies and approached my friends who were in long-term (and loving) relationships or marriages and sought their advice that I started to have more success in this area. That's when I realised for the first time that to get what you want, you have to deserve what you want.

How to say 'no'

Earlier, I spoke about trigger words and how the word 'boring' set me off on an emotional rollercoaster. The experience taught me about trigger words, but my unpleasant reaction could have been completely avoided with one simple word: *No*.

Benjamin Franklin said, 'An ounce of prevention is worth a pound of cure', and I could have easily avoided the uncomfortable situation with my sister by just saying 'no' as soon as the party invitation came in.[3] Nonetheless, saying 'no' is very difficult for most of us. I like to think of saying 'no' as the process of building a muscle. You need to build it over time. The more repetitions you do, the stronger the muscle gets. The more you say 'no', the easier it becomes.

One of the reasons it is so hard to say no is the innate fear of social awkwardness that can come along with it. We as humans have evolved and are wired to want

---

3   From Benjamin Franklin (1983) *Poor Richard's Almanack*. New York: Peter Pauper Press.

to get along with others, and we have an innate need for others to like us.

For thousands of years, we lived as hunter-gatherer tribes, and our survival depended on our ability to get along with others. Like most mental hardwiring, this tendency kept us alive thousands of years ago, but now it just leads to unnecessary anxiety, stress or worry because of our desire to be liked. Psychologists call this tendency 'normative conformity'. Normative conformity is the reason if an old friend invites you for drinks or your boss asks you to take on another job, and you know you are going to struggle to prioritise, the very thought of saying 'no' can still make you feel physically uncomfortable. We feel guilty that if we say 'no' we are going to let somebody else down and potentially damage the relationship we have with them.

For years, every time I was asked to attend social outings or events I really didn't want to go to, I automatically said 'yes'. Then as the date came closer, I would get anxious and stressed. I suffered from stomach ulcers for most of my early twenties, and I attribute a lot of it to the stress of overcommitting myself to things I really didn't want to do.

I've spoken in the 'Trigger words to set you off' section of the book about making rational decisions versus making emotional decisions. Every time I was asked to attend an event, in the moment I always emotionally answered 'yes'. I didn't realise that emotions muddle one's clarity and distract one from the reality of the situation. The fact is that either we can say 'no' and sit in the discomfort for a few minutes or we can say 'yes', only to regret it for days, weeks, months or even years afterwards.

My personality type lends itself to impulsivity. If I were left to my own devices without ever working on my personal development, I would have a 'jump in and think later' approach to nearly everything. This tendency, although having some positives, such as not struggling with taking the first action steps towards new goals, would also cloud my decision-making ability when trying to prioritise what was most important to me. This clouded judgement regularly led me to make emotionally driven decisions where rational choices would have been better options. I got into verbal arguments with friends, had rows with girlfriends and made bad business choices due to this uncontrolled impulsivity, and it is reflected in all areas of my life.

If you have a more rational personality type by nature, then saying 'no' resolutely is enough. But, for those of you who fear the social awkwardness that can emerge from saying 'no' or you need to overcome your desire to please everyone or control your impulsivity or emotions, I'll share some of my strategies for how to say 'no' more effectively.

In Chapter Two, I spoke about the four quadrants – health, wealth, love and fulfilment. Thanks to the four-quadrant system, I find it significantly easier to say 'no' to most things nowadays. Generally, when making any commitment, I ask myself a simple question: 'Is what I'm about to say "yes" to going to move the needle forward in any of the four quadrants?' If the answer is negative, then I just say 'no', resolutely and firmly, end of story. Conversely, if it is going to move the needle forward or potentially open up another door or window of opportunity, then I generally say 'yes'. For me, it's that simple.

Having said that, it took me years to get to this point. Although I hope by the time you finish this book you will be clear about your four quadrants, I also hope these tips and strategies will help tide you over until you've had more practice setting and sticking to your goals for each of them.

Practical tips for saying 'no'

Be it family members, friends or even strangers, it's not easy to say 'no' to people. The following are some practical questions and tips I've used over the years to help me say 'no' to things I really don't want to do.

1. What if it was next Tuesday?

Asking myself the above question is a tactic I implement often. It's easy to commit yourself to things far away in the future – an event, a meeting or even a business project. Although your schedule is busy right now, it looks pretty free in seven weeks, so you agree and say 'yes'. If you do, you've just fallen for the 'planning fallacy'. Just because your schedule looks empty in seven weeks right now, it's unlikely that it's going to be the same when the actual day comes around. It's so far in the future that it feels like another lifetime away.

Still, as the date arrives, you question why you said 'yes' in the first place. One of the strategies I use to get around this is asking the question, 'If this request is for next Tuesday, what will I say?' In most cases, the thought of having to squeeze in another commitment into an already busy schedule makes you realise that you're probably better off saying 'no' to the future commitment. Of course, if it's something you'd love to do this Tuesday, then commit to it. But this is a good tactic for any offers that are for the distant or near-distant future and you're not sure if it's something you would like to do.

2. Refusing without using the word 'no'

I've tried to master this strategy over the years. I'm in a very fortunate position now that I'm normally presented with different opportunities on a weekly or monthly basis. Overwhelmedness is an emotion I have had to tackle over the years, and learning to say 'no' combined with the reframing expression 'I'm so lucky to be drowning in opportunity' is largely how I've dealt with this. This reframing helps me deal with the potential problem of being overwhelmed from being 'too busy' and not appreciating the requests that come my way. Also, as I'm very selective about the projects I work on, I've had to hone the graceful skill of saying 'no' without using the word. I agree with the quote 'Good artists copy; great artists steal', alternately attributed to Pablo Picasso, TS Eliot and others, so feel free to steal the following line from me:

I'm overcommitted at the minute but thank
you so much for thinking of me.

The above line works well for two reasons. One, it helps maintain the relationship with the person who offered you the opportunity as you're expressing that you're flattered they thought of you. Two, it also completely closes off any follow-up for the same request.

If you say, 'I'll get back to you', 'leave it with me' or 'maybe next time', then you'll have to reach out and respond with an inevitable 'no' down the line – or, worse, say 'yes' the next time out of obligation.

If I had a penny for every time I said, 'maybe next time' and then felt obliged when someone reached out a second or third time, I'd have a lot of pennies. Keep your response clean, and you won't feel obligated now or the next time. Also, nearly everyone knows what it's like to be very busy or spread too thin, so most reasonable people will respect that. This way, you're not wasting their time, and they can approach somebody else, knowing exactly where they stand with you.

3. Focus on the opportunity cost

Opportunity cost is the economics term for giving up one thing for another. For example, if you spend money on a bottle of water, you can't spend the same money on a newspaper. You have to say 'no' to one thing so you can say 'yes' to another. The more you think about what you are giving up when you say 'yes', the easier it is to say 'no'.

For instance, I spend a daddy–daughter day with my little girl Holly every week. Nine out of ten times it falls on a Saturday, so I very rarely make other commitments on that day as it is reserved for my daughter. Of course, there are times when I have commitments that fall on a Saturday (then I generally just move our day to Sunday). Realising I am giving up one thing for another and I can't always choose both makes it much easier to say 'no'.

This also comes back to my 'value ladder', discussed in more detail in the next chapter. As my daughter is at the top of the ladder, nothing comes in the way of that relationship. I may move things around, as mentioned above, but I will never start a project or make a life choice where the potential downside affects that relationship. I have spoken earlier in this chapter about making decisions based on the questions, 'What's the upside, what's the downside, and can I handle the potential downside?' If the downside of a decision of mine is that I miss out on the daddy–daughter day as a result of the opportunity cost, then it makes the decision very easy. If you don't know what you want, you will take whatever you get, so get clear on what's valuable and important to you, prioritise those things and say 'no' to the rest.

4. Realise that they don't really care anyway

This was a big realisation for me. For years, I'd get in my head about saying 'no', thinking I'd either burn the bridge in a particular relationship if I didn't attend an event or people would talk negatively about me if I wasn't there. But I'll let you in on a little secret I noticed when I objectively removed myself from most of those situations. The people to whom you said 'no' – they don't really care!

Yes, they may be disappointed initially or even for a few minutes before or during the actual event, especially if your name is brought up in conversation, but guess what happens straight after? Life goes back to normal; they go back to worrying about their own problems, and after a day or two they forget you even said 'no' in the first place.

Except for your inner circle or the five closest people in your life – the people whose opinions truly carry weight – everyone else doesn't care what you do. True, they may have an adverse opinion of you for a brief moment, but then they go back to focusing on themselves and their problems.

Just think about it for a second. Think about a time somebody said 'no' to you or declined an invitation to an event you were holding. Did you spend days or even hours thinking about it and worrying why the person said 'no'? Probably not. More likely, you spent a couple of minutes wondering about it and then went back to your thoughts, worries or daily routines. Sometimes, objectively taking ourselves out of a given situation and realising how we will feel if the figurative shoe were on the other foot allows us to realise how we would react in the same situation. Generally, as soon as you do this you tend to stop feeling bad about saying 'no'.

It's also worth noting that this objectivity works in nearly every situation. There's an old saying that you can sometimes miss the entire forest if you're staring directly at a single tree. So remove yourself from any given situation, look at it objectively, rationally or from the vantage point of the other person, and you will realise that saying 'no' isn't as big of a deal as you made it out to be in your head.

I can make promises about only a few things in this life. But I promise that if you get better at saying 'no' and focus on saying 'yes' to the most important things for you and move the needle forward in your life, goals or relationships, you will be significantly happier. If you don't live life on your terms, you will live it on someone else's; and as someone who did that for years, I'm telling you it is a recipe for misery.

Becoming indifferent

As you continue to own everything aimed at your direction, separate the wheat from the chaff and absorb any golden messages that may lie in an insult, you will become increasingly indifferent to others' opinions of you.

When you focus on your journey, running your race or having your ladder against the right wall, you stop going through life with the goal of gaining approval or disapproval. As you are indifferent to others' opinions, you will feel no sting if insults are aimed at you. I am the embodiment of your mess becoming your message as this held me back for so long.

I wanted to start my own business since I was nineteen years old, but I was afraid of what my friends and family members would think. I didn't dare to start until five years later, and even at the age of twenty-four, I still worried about what people would say if I failed. I was so scared the people I knew would laugh at me for leaving a secure, well-paying teaching job to start a fitness business from scratch.

To make matters worse, I would make decisions based on the opinions of others – people who knew nothing about business or even fitness in most cases. You can only bang your head against the wall so often before you start wondering why it's hurting. If what you're doing right now isn't helping you move closer to your end goal, then why are you doing it? If you have a headache, you can take a painkiller or even bandage your head up, but wouldn't it be easier just to stop banging it against the wall in the first place? My metaphorical headbanging was constantly looking for others' opinions on what I should do.

I realised that my tendency to seek others' opinions was directly correlated to my lack of confidence. If I wasn't sure about what I wanted, I asked fifty people for their opinions on what I should do, and my goals never got any clearer. On the other hand, when making any decisions today, be it related to business, fitness or my personal life, I ask two or three people in my inner circle, generally mentors or people who are best suited to offer advice. After that, I contemplate the potential upsides, downsides and my ability to handle the downsides, and then I make the decision and commit to it fully. This strategy may sound simple, but it took me nearly a decade to get to this point. I hope reading this will greatly shorten your learning curve. As I said earlier, you have to learn from mistakes, but they don't have to be your mistakes. Feel free to learn from mine.

Remember, the higher the number of people whose opinion you seek, the less confident you are in what you're doing. The answer isn't to ask more people; it's to get clearer on your target or end goal and then ask for advice from the people who can help get you there. Do you want to drop a few dress sizes or get a six-pack? Cool, set that target or goal, make it clear in your mind and then go find the people who know how to get you there. Do you want to get a better job or start your company around what you're passionate about? Cool, set that target or goal, make it clear in your mind and then go find the people who know how to get you there.

You may be thinking, 'But I don't know anyone who can help get me there'. I didn't either at first, but reframe that question to 'I haven't found the person who can get me there ... yet!' and see how quickly your reticular activation system, your brain's internal GPS or the metaphysical law of attraction starts to kick in. As the Theosophist saying goes, 'When the student is ready, the teacher will appear'.

Nothing changes until you make a decision. It is

paramount that you are clear about your target or end goal and then make sure your action steps map onto your ambition. I'm not saying that you specifically have to get in great shape, earn more money or have fulfilling personal relationships. That may not be what you want. Your mission may be completely different. You may want to become a professional actor, sports star or musician, and that's great too. If that's the case, then set that as your goal.

In the next section, I discuss my last tactic to stop caring about what people think of you, which I learned from a neighbour's dog.

Barking-dog strategy

Have you ever knocked at a door only to hear a frantic dog barking at you from the other side? How about a stray dog or even a domesticated one as you approach its territory? What happened? It probably started hysterically barking at you. How long did that situation bother you? Did you spend the next three days wondering why the dog barked at you or thinking you were a bad person because of the incident? Did you question all the decisions you made in life up until the point because the dog barked at you? Probably not. Then why do we do that when people aim negativity, unsupportive criticisms or insults in our direction?

This last strategy to deal with insults or negativity is the 'barking-dog' strategy. Before I achieved clarity on who is in my inner circle and the five people whose opinion mattered, I created the barking-dog strategy to help me navigate through the world with reduced insecurity. On the days I'm not feeling very mentally strong, I always go back to this technique.

I like to think of the insults from other people like the barking of a dog. When a dog barks, you may make a mental note that it dislikes you, but it would be stupid to allow yourself to become upset by it, to go through the whole day thinking 'Oh, dear! That dog doesn't like me', yet we do this all the time with people.

As I started to understand people better, notice the ungodly amount of projection (people putting their insecurities onto others to make themselves feel better) they inflict and observe how often I actually did the same, I learned how unsupportive that approach was.

I treat the negative comments aimed at my direction the same way I treat the barking of a dog. If I don't let a dog's barking annoy or upset me, then why would I waste my mental energy on negative words and comments or give them the power to affect me?

The reason I still use the barking-dog strategy is to get better at dealing with negativity, unsupportive criticisms or insults, and the strategy is a lot like showering. If you shower today, you'll feel clean, but you need to do it every day (or at least several times a week) or else your body will get dirty again. Your mental strength is no different. If you don't stay on top of it every day and apply the strategies that work for you, then it won't stay strong. One of my sports coaches once told me, 'If you *stay* ready, you don't have to *get* ready', and I've carried that advice with me to this day.

Hearing a comment, you won't be able to flick a switch and suddenly stop caring about what people think of you. That's not how it works, but treat it like a dog's barking and you will feel a little better the first time, a little bit mentally stronger the next time, and so on. Building your mental strength is a lot like building a wall. You can set out to build the biggest and best wall ever created, but that's not how it gets built. You build it brick by brick. You lay the first brick as perfectly as a brick can be laid, and then you place the next brick on top of it. Do this every day, and soon you'll have a wall. Start building your 'mental-strength wall' today. The next time you receive negativity, unsupportive criticisms or insults from people you don't know or care about, remember the words aimed at you are exactly like the barks of a stray dog. Woof, woof.

5

Rewire Self-Sabotage

The reason I'm so big on deserving what one wants is because of my issues with self-sabotage over the years. In my early and mid-twenties, I would work so hard towards a goal, but as soon as I achieved it I would self-sabotage as I didn't feel I deserved it. After hitting my body fat target, I would binge on ice cream for three weeks. I would meet an amazing woman, spend weeks courting her but get afraid she'd leave me, and break up with her before she could.

The fear of failure knocks down a lot of people, and I discuss this in the 'Rewire Failure As Feedback' chapter, but the fear of success destroys just as many opportunities. We're just generally less aware of it as it normally manifests at a subconscious level.

In 2016, when I first started making good money, I couldn't spend it fast enough! I bought a new car, attended expensive seminars, redid my wardrobe and bought a fancy watch, all because I subconsciously felt unworthy of having money. Looking back, I didn't feel like I deserved it. Of course, at the time, I didn't understand the reasons for my behaviour, but then I heard about the theory of the 'financial thermometer'.

The idea is that you are conformable having a certain amount of money in your bank account, normally what you're used to having or what you grew up seeing as your baseline. If you are conformable with having X amount of money in your bank account, as soon as it goes up to Y amount, you spend it (normally needlessly); and on the flip side, if it goes down to Z amount, you curb your spending until it gets back to an amount you are conformable with.

For argument's sake, let's say having £5,000 in your bank account is your financial thermometer marking. Your current account goes slightly above or slightly below this depending on the time of the month, but it's normally within striking distance of this figure. If you suddenly win or inherit another £5,000, what will you do? You buy new clothes, go on holiday or redo the house, and that £5,000 is normally gone within a couple of months. Why couldn't you just leave it in your account? Did you need new clothes? Would you have gone on holiday otherwise? Did you really need to redo the house right now? Again, all are pertinent questions, and why you do something is normally more important than what you actually do. If you felt the money was burning a hole in your pocket and you were spending your free time wondering how you were going to spend it, your financial thermometer was likely set to a certain point and you needed to get it back to baseline. It will regulate itself automatically if you don't do something to change it.

The same applies to weight gain and body composition. Even after you take into consideration the downregulation of certain hormones contributing to weight gain or body compositional change, a considerable part of your self-destructive behaviour comes down to your subconscious self-sabotaging because you feel unworthy of what you're getting. For example, if you're trying to drop three dress sizes or develop abs for the first time, but you don't feel like you deserve to look a certain way, it's unlikely you're going to keep that weight off in the long term. Once you do the groundwork and realise a lot of your self-sabotaging is on a subconscious level, then bringing it to your awareness is the first step towards fixing it. On the bright side, there is a very simple antidote to the self-sabotage disease: owning what you've done to this point and then taking action to deserve what you want going forward. As the famous Chinese proverb goes, 'The best time to plant a tree was twenty years ago; the next best time is today'.

I'm an advocate of going through struggles and moving outside of your comfort zone because deserving what you want and believing you've earned it make keeping it when you actually get it easier. Building the discipline to do the right things every day allows you to tough it out one inch at a time. Regardless of how slowly you go or how slowly you improve, as long as your ladder is against the right wall you'll get everything you want along the way and won't have to take two steps back for each step forward.

As billionaire investor Charlie Munger puts it, 'Step by step you get ahead, but not necessarily in fast spurts. But you build discipline by preparing for fast spurts... Slug it out one inch at a time, day by day. At the end of the day – if you live long enough – most people get what they deserve.'[1]

Hooking up with someone 'way out of your league'

Do you know what happens when you get what you want and don't feel you deserve it? You will self-sabotage until it goes away. For example, there may have been a time when you were dating someone who you perceived to be way out of your league. When you feel you don't deserve something, just watch how your behaviour changes. In this case, it normally manifests in one of two extreme ways.

The first way is being overly affectionate by showering the other person with excessive amounts of gifts or attention, which can come across as needy and push the other person away. The second way is feeling insecure and jealous easily and pushing the other person away through your projected insecurity and irrational behaviour. And what makes the behaviour worse?

---

1   C Munger and P D Kaufman (2005) *Poor Charlie's Almanack*. Missouri: Walsworth Publishing Company.

Rationalising it! You'll create a story around it and say, 'They were probably out of my league anyway', thus making the breakup a self-fulfilled prophecy.

Another bitter pill to swallow is that they may not have been out of your league in the first place. They might have had a completely different set of values as to what they wanted in a relationship, but you used your own value metrics, past experiences or perspective to determine what made you worthy in their eyes.

Here's an example to explain my above point, and apologies in advance for scoring vanity metrics such a looks on a 1–10 scale, but I think it helps to illustrate my point.

You start seeing someone who is sweet, funny and has a good respectable job or social status, and who is also a solid 10/10 in the looks department. Of course, everyone has their own idea of what makes someone a 10/10, but for this example imagine that they are your version of a 10/10. Now you, on the other hand, rate yourself as a 7/10 on a good day; some days, you feel like you're higher, sometimes lower. You think you are definitely somewhat attractive but certainly not a 10/10.

Let's also say you value physical attractiveness as one of the most important qualities in a potential partner, so you have put this person on a pedestal straight away. You assume because you value physical attractiveness highly, everyone else does too. In psychology, that's called a 'false-consensus effect' or 'false-consensus bias', whereby people tend to over-estimate the extent to which their opinions, beliefs, preferences, values and habits are normal and typical of those of others.[2] Basically, you think that because physical attractiveness is important to you it must be the same for others. You can replace physical attractiveness with any other trait – such as social status, intelligence or sense of humour – in this example.

As you think the person you're seeing is out of your league, you start to change your behaviour to match your insecurities; thus, the unravelling begins.

There's a good chance that this has happened to you at some stage or to a friend or family member who was perceived to be 'punching above their weight'. What if I told you this is an opinion, not a fact? Yes, that person may be a 10/10 to you, but looks may not necessarily be the highest priority on their value ladder.

Value ladder

I briefly mentioned the value ladder earlier, but here it is in all its glory. Let's look at the value ladder in terms of a romantic relationship. It's worth noting that the case is the same for personal and familial relationships, too, just the metrics of what is important may be very different. For example, you may not care at all about the looks of your best friend, but having a best friend who is a good listener or has the ability to carry on stimulating conversations may be very important to you.

---

2   J Krueger and R W Clement (1995) 'The Truly False Consensus
     Effect: An ineradicable and egocentric bias in social perception',
     J Pers Soc Psychol, Apr; 68(4): 579.

Before I continue, I just want to say that I am not a relationship expert or certified counsellor; the romantic value ladder example below is merely a means to illustrate some of the psychological misjudgements that we all make. To deserve what you want, you have to be clear on the things that may be holding you back in achieving your goal.

With that in mind, let's say your romantic value ladder is as follows, with the most important metric at the top and the least important at the bottom:

1. Physical attractiveness and looks
2. Sense of humour and ability to make you laugh
3. Intelligence and the ability to have a stimulating conversation
4. Income, job security, social status, etc

Once the false-consensus bias kicks in, you assume that everyone else has a similar order to their value ladder as yours. Nonetheless, picture for a minute that the person you are seeing has a value ladder like this one:

1. Sense of humour and ability to make you laugh
2. Income, job security, social status, etc
3. Intelligence and the ability to have a stimulating conversation
4. Physical attractiveness and looks

The person you're seeing holds the values of sense of humour and job security at the top of their ladder, and they aren't actually concerned about how good-looking their partner is. Physical attractiveness is actually at the bottom of their value ladder! Yet you self-sabotaged a perfectly good relationship or made up a story around it because you didn't look at it objectively. If you have ever seen a rich middle-aged gentleman of high social status and a stunning young woman together, then this illustrates the value ladder point perfectly. This is obviously an extreme example, but it shows you how *different people value different things*. Once you rewire your thinking to avoid self-sabotage, achieving your goals gets much easier from there as the compound effect starts to kick in.

To get what you want, you have to deserve what you want

The questions you ask yourself are very powerful and switching my question from 'How do I get a better partner' to 'How do I deserve a better partner?' opened my mind to a completely new way of thinking. Getting a better partner is external, as it puts the focus on the other person and what characteristics or attributes this other person needs to have for me to be attracted to them.

Yes, it is important to know what you value in another person. To get what you want, you need to know exactly what it is that you want. Yet, this way of thinking takes the agency away from you. It's an easy option. You don't really have to do anything as it's not up to you anymore. We have all done it, including me. You're effectively leaving it up to the traditional 'luck' defined as success or failure apparently brought by chance rather than one's actions.

I've long been a believer that 'luck is when preparation meets opportunity'. Changing the question to 'How do I deserve a better partner?' allows you to own your fate and change whatever you need to in order to prepare yourself for when the opportunity arises. The opportunity will come; it's just up to you to recognise it when it does show up. This goes for everything in your life. How do I deserve a better body? I make healthier food choices and exercise more. How do I deserve more money? I provide higher-quality services to more people or become so valuable that people pay me extremely well for what I do.

Regardless of whether you believe that the universe conspires to give you everything you want or in the cognitive neuroscience of your reticular activation system – your brain's internal GPS, which we'll address as part of the discussion on 'tuned perception' in the 'Rewire Goal Setting' chapter – this strategy works. Once you know your target or goal and put yourself in the best situation to receive it, when the opportunity comes, you can grab it with both hands.

6

The Compound Effect

One of my favourite stories in *Aesop's Fables* is 'The Tortoise and the Hare', where the tortoise beats the hare by slowly putting one foot in front of the other and never getting distracted from the end goal, while the hare ruins its chance of winning the race by looking for shortcuts and quick fixes. The tale teaches us that 'slow and steady wins the race'.

This is pretty good advice for real life, and although there is definitely a time to go fast, I love the tale so much because of my issues with patience and my past tendency to constantly give in to immediate gratification in nearly everything I did. I used to be the human embodiment of the hare. I wanted everything right now and would take any shortcut or quick fix to get to the end goal faster. I bought every single supplement on the market that promised to make me 'muscular and ripped'. I was attracted to 'get-rich-quick' courses, classes and seminars because I thought one could make a lot of money from them. Although I empathise deeply with people who have a similar default disposition, this approach is completely wrong!

All successful people I spoke to – the men and women in great shape, the millionaire entrepreneurs, or the couples in loving and thriving relationships – preached the same thing: No silver-bullet diet, investment or marriage strategy exists that will bring success. Being successful is about doing a lot of small and simple things, but here's the kicker – it's about doing them consistently over time and then letting what's called the compound effect take its course.

Over the past decade, one of the personality traits I have done the most work on improving is patience. As I mentioned above, my default mode is instant gratification. I generally want this shiny toy, that piece of cake or those defined abs right now. This impatience, born out of insecurity and a desire to fill a gap with something external or material, never served me well. Then, things changed when I learned about the compound effect.

Compounding is a term used in money investment circles to refer to an exponential increase in the value of an investment due to the earning interest on both the principal (what you invested initially) and accumulated interest (what you earn over time). Investing is basically getting free money. The billionaire tycoon Warren Buffett calls it the 'secret to great wealth', and the genius Nobel Laureate Albert Einstein called compounding 'the eighth wonder of the world'.

Compounding doesn't just work in finance or physics; everything you do compounds over time. The food you eat, the exercise you do, the choices you make – they all compound.

How has the compound effect impacted you?

Think about how compounding has affected your life so far. Your food choices over the past three, six or twelve months (or even years in some cases) have had a significant effect on your body composition and energy levels. One doesn't put on weight or get out of shape by making one poor food decision. It does not even happen over a day of bad eating. Consistently making food choices that are not aligned with your goal of being leaner or fitter has led to the problem of not being in the shape you desire. If you do this for weeks, months or years, the problem compounds. Bad habits compound! The upside is that good habits compound just as easily.

Everything you do can have a compound effect – your exercise regimen, your morning or nightly routines, your way of spending your free time, even your company. All of them compound over time and become hardwired habits. Good or bad, we are what we consistently do, and all our good habits and bad habits compound over time. That, my friend, is the compound effect.

I first learned of the compound effect and the impact of my habits on my life when I was in my early twenties. At the time, I was working full time as a primary school teacher in London, and I had little to no money in savings and wasn't in the best place in any area of my life. Broke and unfulfilled, I lived in a constant state of worry and anxiety.

I used to get up every morning after setting seven alarms (so I could snooze six times). After waking up, I would rush out the door and commute an hour and a half to the school where I worked, all the while staring out the train window or keeping my head down listening to music. I would get to work, have some food, grab a cup of coffee, set up my class for the morning session, teach, work through the day (and through lunchtime in most cases) and finish about an hour after the kids left. After that, I would go home, flop down in front of the TV to watch game shows or sports news, have some chocolate, fall asleep on the couch, wake up, talk with my housemates for a while, pack my lunch for the next day and then go to bed. I did this on autopilot for nearly two years.

At the time, I never once thought about what I was doing. If I'm honest, although I liked my job, I spent the weekdays counting down until the weekend. Every Friday, I was ecstatic about sleeping in the next morning, and every Sunday evening, I would feel a wave of anxiety hit me about all the things I had to do the following week. I called these feelings 'Friday ecstasy' and 'Sunday blues'.

When I started my fitness business, my primary goal, other than making enough money to live, was never to have those feelings again. Those Sunday blues felt like mild depression hitting me every week, and I didn't want to feel that way anymore. Nowadays, I never even realise what day it is, and I love Sunday evenings as I know I'm going to have an amazing week ahead. I equally love Fridays because I normally get to have a movie night with my daughter or meet someone in my inner circle for dinner. Every day in between is just as great. This is an example of 'What you focus your mind on is what will expand'. When you are clear about how you want your day, your week or even your life to be, you can start manifesting it into reality.

I'm also very grateful for the Sunday blues as, without the contrast, it wouldn't be possible to do what I do now. There is no good without bad, no light without darkness, no success without failure. Remember, everything is how you choose to see it.

If you are living through your version of Sunday blues right now – you may be out of shape or overweight, broke and bordering on welfare, in a toxic relationship you're not sure you want to stay in – all those bad times will give you a stronger reference or contrast point when you come out the other side. The bad times make you grateful for the good times. Embrace them as they're normally the fuel that sparks the fire for change.

We do so many things on autopilot, not even realising we're doing them. Only after living on autopilot for two years did I realise something had to change. In my first book, *The Fitness Mindset*, I discussed my catalyst for change, the moment I realised I wasn't doing what I was meant to be doing with my life. My trigger moment happened when I was listening to an audiobook of Stephen R Covey's *7 Habits of Highly Effective People* while walking down a dark street in East London.[1]

In the book, Covey talks about imagining oneself going to the funeral of a loved one. Picture yourself driving to the funeral parlour, parking the car and getting out. As you enter the building, you notice the flowers and hear the organ music. You see the faces of friends and family passing along the way. When you walk down to the front of the room and look inside the coffin, you suddenly come face to face with yourself. This is *your* funeral, three years from today. All the people have come to honour you, to express love and appreciation for your life. While you wait for the service to begin, you see four speakers. The first is someone from your family – a child, parent, aunt, uncle, niece or nephew. The second is one of your friends, someone who knew you closely as a person. The third is from your work or profession, and the fourth is someone you were involved with from your community. Now think deeply. What would you like each of these speakers to say about you and your life?

This section struck me more than anything else in the entire book.

The picture painted in my mind was so clear and

I   S Covey (1989) *The 7 Habits of Highly Effective People.* New York: Simon & Schuster.

vivid that it hit me like a ton of bricks. It also dawned on me that I wasn't happy with the answer forming in my head when I asked myself what the speakers would say about me. That was the moment I decided to leave London to pursue my passion. Shortly after, I left my job, moved back home with my parents (broke and on welfare) and tried to set up a new life that mattered. I decided to finally get my ladder against the right wall.

However, I was also aware that I needed to make new choices and form some new habits. You don't decide your future; you decide your habits, and your habits decide your future. All this time, I had been either making unsupportive decisions that moved me further away from my end goal or been led by ones made on autopilot, and the compound effect had been working against me. I decided then and there that something had to change. New thoughts lead to new decisions. New decisions lead to new actions. New actions lead to new habits. New habits lead to new results.

The payoff of the compound effect

The compound effect is the principle of reaping tremendous rewards from a series of seemingly small and insignificant choices. What's most interesting about the process is that even though the results are massive, the steps, at the moment, don't feel that earth-shattering. It's like my earlier analogy of building a wall and the importance of laying each brick as perfectly as possible.

Something as incredible as the Great Wall of China started with a single brick. We see this momentous human-made wall that boggles the mind, but it started with a brick and then another and then another. Every time my self-talk starts clouding my mind with unsupportive stories like 'You can't run that distance', 'You can't lift that weight', 'You can't write that book' or 'You're not good enough or smart enough to do that; it's just too big', I think of the Great Wall of China. I normally follow it with the reminder that 'ordinary things done consistently well lead to extraordinary results'.

I am still plagued by negative thoughts when trying to achieve a big goal or hit a new target. I normally repeat those words or write them down until those unsupportive thoughts disappear and my focus switches back to WIN – What's Important Now – figuratively laying whatever brick is in front of me.

Don't focus on the massive goal or target you have set yourself; instead, focus on what you need to do right now that feeds the goal. Don't focus on all the weight you want to lose; rather, focus on getting your next meal right or your next workout complete. Don't focus on the time it will take to build a loving relationship; focus on being present for your next interaction. Tell me what you focus on, and I will tell you what's going to expand.

Whether you're using this strategy for improving your fitness, health, relationships or finances, the changes are subtle as there's no big massive payoff in one go. For years, I always looked for the silver-bullet supplement that would make me bigger or leaner. I searched for the one course or book that would make me rich. I would ask people in relationships for the one thing I needed to do to find the right romantic partner. These were instances of asking the wrong questions and seeing things the wrong way. As I talked to more successful people – I'm defining 'successful people' as those who were in the positions I strived to replicate or model – a pattern started to form in my mind.

True, there are people out there who will try to sell you the single big thing that will change your entire life with the snap of a finger, but when I searched deeper I found something else. The advice that seemed to stand the test of time was nearly identical across all the successful people I spoke with. It may be worded in a slightly different way, but the principle has always remained the same: It's not about the one thing you do that gets you to your goals; it's what you do consistently over time.

There isn't one single diet or exercise regimen that gets you in great shape. If there was, everybody would follow it, and everyone would look the way they wanted. It's about the cumulative effect of making better decisions consistently over time and making sure they're aligned with your end goals. As someone who has worked as a fitness professional for years, getting in shape is about consistently getting the fundamentals right – eating a calorie-surplus diet if you want to gain weight, eating a calorie-deficit diet if you want to lose weight or reduce body fat and following a training programme that supports your end goal.

For example, if you want to become bigger or stronger, it helps to focus on your compound lifts in the gym – squat, bench and deadlift. If you want to get fitter: run, cycle or swim more often. Then, if you have all of that right, add in some supplements that can potentially speed up your progress. As a fitness professional, I saw the world through that particular lens and applied those lessons to other areas of my life. I now know for a fact that there is no such thing as a 'silver-bullet fat-loss supplement'; yet, earlier in my life, I was always looking for the next big supplement that would just 'melt fat off my body'.

In hindsight, my attempts were ridiculous. Success leaves clues, and if I had asked anybody with whom I would have traded positions, they would have told me that finding success is doing all the right things consistently well over time. I didn't ask them; my mindset was wrong. I wanted the easy answer. I wanted the quick fix. Truly, I didn't need a silver-bullet supplement; I needed a mindset change. I had to fix my mindset before I could change anything else.

Getting in shape is a great example of the compound effect. When I started following the advice of other fitness professionals, it felt like nothing was happening at first. I was consistently eating the right foods for my body, training regularly on a programme specific to my goals and adding in supplements that sped up the progress. But until a month or two had passed, I did not notice any changes. From that point onwards, they became more pronounced every month. In a year and a half, I went from a normal gymgoer who worked full time as a teacher to a professional fitness model who was sponsored to travel the world to compete in bodybuilding shows.

Your end goal may not be to become a professional fitness model or a bodybuilder. To be honest, as I recounted in the section titled 'Anxiety' in *The Fitness Mindset*, that lifestyle isn't all it's cracked up to be, but that was my end goal at the time. Although that lifestyle didn't lend itself to helping me become the person I wanted to be once my daughter was born, it served to add a very strong leg to my confidence table. It also gave me a strong reference point when it came to the compound effect. I've since been taking the same principles and applying them to my new fitness goals, personal relationships and business ventures.

As I mentioned earlier, you build confidence by saying you're going to do something and then going and doing it. I have chosen to share my fitness example because when I made the switch to start my own business, the exact same recipe for success kept coming back to me. Yes, I tried the 'get-rich-quick' schemes and building a 'money-making sales funnel' and all the other propaganda that gets peddled to misinformed twenty-year-olds; but as with fitness, the more people I talked to, the more I realised they weren't the path to success.

Building a business is a lot like building your body. Instead of spending time in the gym, you spend time finding ways to improve the lives of other people. Instead of researching the best foods for your body, you research better ways to advertise or market your service or product. When I realised that success left clues, I modelled the behaviour of the people who I thought were successful. It wasn't easy because I still had to cultivate the right habits and let them compound, but the recipe for success really is that simple.

What are you doing on autopilot?

Here's a question to ask yourself: What am I doing right now that is on autopilot?

It may be your eating habits, your workout regimen, your job or your relationship, but what are you just letting happen to you and are not consciously aware of? Take thirty seconds to think about it. What part of your life or quadrant is on autopilot that you are trying to improve?

I ask myself this question every month and apply it to my four quadrants – health, wealth, love and fulfilment. Sometimes, the answers are positive. For example, my food choices are largely automatic and are on autopilot now. I know what foods work for my body, give me energy and fuel me for the day. As I feel much better when I avoid artificial ingredients and processed food, I try and stick to mostly whole foods, which include different fruits and vegetables. I never really think about my food choices anymore.

Other times, certain habits or tendencies may start to compound negatively, and I have to catch them before they become more difficult to change. For example, while writing this book I found myself disconnecting or switching off while conversing with friends and family members. My mind would wander to the chapter I had written the day before or what I was going to write the following morning, and I would zone out of conversations. Again, it's easy to tell yourself the story, 'It's only for a short period; the book will be finished soon'. But once you start letting yourself off the hook for small things, the tendency will spill over into the bigger things. Amidst a conversation with somebody, if your mind has ever wandered somewhere else – to a work task, a fight with your partner, an upcoming meeting, etc – then you're familiar with this experience.

In such instances, to break the cycle, I normally have to verbally acknowledge that my mind was somewhere else and apologise for it. That's enough to bring my attention back to focus. Now, I'm not saying you have to do the same, but for me, nurturing my relationships with the people in my inner circle is important, and I try and look out for small things that affect those relationships. As that's what I want to compound over time, I try and make sure my actions map onto my ambition.

A lot of people tend to underestimate the significance

of creating the right habits and miss how dramatically the compound effect can impact things over time. For instance, they quit after eight days of running or going to the gym because they're still overweight, or they quit playing the piano after three months because they don't sound anything like Beethoven.

What they fail to realise is that it is these small, seemingly insignificant steps that compound over time. When I worked as a personal fitness trainer, I would set up a consultation prior to undertaking any new clients. I often worked with overweight or out-of-shape people who had taken up some radical bar or juice diet. You know, the diets that make the promise that you will lose a lot of weight in a very short period but massively restrict how much you eat during that period. Yes, those ones.

Anyway, we would sit down, and they would tell me that they were 50 lbs overweight and wanted to lose it all in the next month. First, yes, it is possible to lose 50 lbs in a month, especially if you're morbidly obese to start with. You can lose considerable weight by overly restricting calorie intake and drastically lowering carbohydrate and water intake. This practice is not safe, and I do not recommend it to anyone, but it can be done. But is it sustainable? No. Such scenarios always remind me of the old Chinese proverb: 'The wall that goes up quickly, falls down quickly'.

If you have been out of shape or overweight for years, you're not going to lose all those kilos in a few weeks and keep them off over the long term. The reason you're overweight or out of shape now is normally down to the choices you've made up to this point. Again, they may have been conscious or misinformed choices or those simply made on autopilot, but they were made. If you're overweight because you have been making poor food choices, that's fine, but own it. Once you own it, it's back in your control, and you can change it. The same principle applies to your job choices, relationships or finances. If you've been making the wrong choices, don't blame anybody else as it's not their fault; and even if it were, will blaming others help you move forward? Others are not going to change your life; only you can. Regardless of where you are right now, what's important is where you're going. Don't ignore the reality; don't make up excuses or create stories about it.

I once had a client called Julie who was three stone over her ideal weight. She had tried every bar, juice and fad diet, and, at thirty-three years of age, she had been dieting nearly half her adult life. Despite all the years spent dieting, she was still no closer to a healthy weight. Again, as I mentioned earlier, the definition of 'insanity' is 'doing the same thing over and over again and expecting a different result'. If you have been dieting most of your adult life and are still unhappy with how you look, it's time to change something. Remember, it's better to be at the bottom of the ladder against the right wall than at the top of the ladder against the wrong wall. In this case, you may get to the top of the wrong ladder and lose that weight by crash dieting, but that ladder is going to come crashing down as soon as you start eating normal food again, and you're going to find yourself exactly where you started – at the bottom.

When I sat down with Julie, she told me her backstory and that her goal was to lose 50 lbs in the next three weeks so she could attend a family event. I listened to everything she had to say and then told her that she could potentially lose 50 lbs in three weeks, but there was no way she was going to be able to keep that weight off over the long term.

The truth was that she needed to rewire her mindset, make better food choices and find an exercise regimen that she could stick to, and I explained all this to her. I told her that if she was going to work with me, she wasn't going to have the massive weight fluctuations anymore. We were going to find systems and strategies that worked for her lifestyle and schedule and that would help her to lose weight the right way by gradually reducing her calorie intake and making healthier food choices. The goal was to keep her energy levels high as her training or exercise volume gradually increased.

As I discussed her exercise and diet plan with Julie, I noticed her starting to frown at me. She didn't look very happy. Then, she asked, 'How long will all *that* take?' and I replied, 'To lose 50 lbs, keep it off and continue to reduce your body fat even further the right way, probably about three months'. She countered with a sentiment I've heard over a thousand times while working as a personal trainer: 'Three months? But that's so much time!'

My answer, which became an inside joke among all my clients, was: 'Well, the time is going to pass anyway'. I told her she could keep following the 'yo-yo' diets and let her weight go up and down like a roller-coaster or she could finally get the right plan in place, get her ladder up against the right wall and finally start climbing it. She signed up on the spot.

Time is going to pass anyway

One of the most unsupportive stories we can let churn in our heads is: 'It's going to take way too much time'. Before I go on, yes, there are times when it makes sense to completely cut the cord on something and it's smarter to redirect your focus elsewhere or take into consideration the opportunity cost of what else you could do with that time and energy. But the cut-the-cord approach is not helpful when it comes to things that can run in parallel with your life – things you can maintain at the same time: your health, your fitness, your relationships and your job. Being happy or successful in one area can improve the happiness and success in the other areas.

The reason the four quadrants idea works so well for people is that it's not designed as a 'first this, then that' approach – first I'll get the job I want, then I'll get into good shape, or first I'll start a company, then I'll find an amazing romantic partner. They can run in parallel. You can do them at the same time!

Yes, it's easy and even tempting to find a quick fix or succumb to instant gratification, resorting to the bar or juice diet, the 'get-rich-quick' scheme or whatever your figurative silver bullet is. I completely understand this, and we do it because we think it will get us where we want to be even faster or will make things easier. Remember, if you do what is easy, your life will be hard, and if something sounds too good to be true, it probably is.

I will let you in on a little secret, though. The 'get-it-quickly method' is actually the 'get-it-slowly method'. As you take one step forward – lose weight quickly or earn extra cash – you'll have to take two steps backwards; your weight rebounds or you lose the trust of the people with whom you did business, and now you're in a worse position than when you started. Try compounding that over time and see where it gets you!

I'm not a mathematician, but 'one step forward and two steps backwards' leaves you in a worse position than when you started. If you think that the alternative will take too much time, just remember that time is going to pass anyway. You may as well spend it making supportive choices, getting your ladder against the right wall and doing all the things you want that work in parallel with each other.

If you're not sure how to do that, go find the people

who have already done it and ask them. There's no such thing as a new problem. The solution is out there, and you just have to go and find it. I'm telling you exactly what I did in the hope it becomes the catalyst for your future success in whatever is important to you. I made the same mistakes over and over again, but please be smarter than me and don't chase quick fixes. Time is going to pass anyway, so spend it doing things the right way. The tortoise in *Aesop's Fables* and the people who built the Great Wall of China knew it, too. You win the race step by step, and you build a wall brick by brick. You can do neither all at once.

The magic penny

Just to give you an idea of the power of compounding, here's one of my favourite examples called 'the magic penny'. Darren Hardy's book *The Compound Effect* provides several examples of the power of compounding, but the magic penny is probably my favourite. The scenario goes like this: If you were given a choice to receive $1 million in one month or a penny that doubled every day for thirty days, which would you choose?

When I first read the question, I knew the penny that doubled every day must be the better choice as it sounded like a trick question. Though, how much better it would be was something I didn't realise immediately. The following is the calculation for the penny doubling every day:

1. Day 1: $0.01
2. Day 2: $0.02
3. Day 3: $0.04
4. Day 4: $0.08
5. Day 5: $0.16
6. Day 6: $0.32
7. Day 7: $0.64
8. Day 8: $1.28
9. Day 9: $2.56
10. Day 10: $5.12
11. Day 11: $10.24
12. Day 12: $20.48
13. Day 13: $40.96
14. Day 14: $81.92
15. Day 15: $163.84
16. Day 16: $327.68
17. Day 17: $655.36
18. Day 18: $1,310.72
19. Day 19: $2,621.44
20. Day 20: $5,242.88
21. Day 21: $10,485.76
22. Day 22: $20,971.52
23. Day 23: $41,943.04
24. Day 24: $83,886.08
25. Day 25: $167,772.16
26. Day 26: $335,544.32
27. Day 27: $671,088.64
28. Day 28: $1,342,177.28
29. Day 29: $2,684,354.56
30. Day 30: $5,368,709.12

The difference is quite significant. The amounts remain small until day 18; then, the growth is dramatic.

The above example shows you the power of compounding in the investment world, but let's see how compounding works in an everyday scenario.

Let's take three friends who grew up together. They're all married and live in the same town. They also have very similar backgrounds, intelligence levels and personalities. Each makes about £50,000 a year. They each have an average health and body weight composition, plus a little bit of that dreaded 'marriage flab'.

Linda, friend number one, plods along in life, doing what she's always done. She's happy, or thinks she is, but regularly complains that nothing ever really changes or improves in her life.

Sarah, friend number two, starts making some small and seemingly inconsequential positive changes in her life. She begins reading a chapter of a personal development book or listening to an audiobook for thirty minutes every day on her commute to work. She's turned her car into a library on wheels. She wants to improve her life but doesn't want to make a fuss about it and doesn't want to do anything too drastic. She chooses to make some simple changes that can improve her life. An article she recently read informed her that cutting 125 calories from her diet every day might help her lose a bit of fat around her tummy. I'm talking 125 calories from day one, not gradually decreasing it every day. Just a one-off decision. No big deal. That means cutting down a cup of cereal in the morning or trading a can of soda for water at lunchtime. She's also decided to take the stairs at work from now on and skip using the lift. Again, a very simple change, something most people can do. She is determined to stick with these choices, knowing that even though they're simple, she can easily be tempted to abandon them.

A study conducted at the University of London reports that it takes sixty-six days to form a new habit.[2] Sarah has made the commitment that the changes are non-negotiable – she's doing them whether she feels like it or not, and this is something that successful people do. It doesn't matter how small or big, but if you make a commitment, then stick to it whether you feel like it or not. Sometimes, small changes are actually easier to abandon than the big ones. It's easy to make up a story like 'Sure, it's only one can of soda' or 'I'm tired today; I'll take the elevator', and before you know it, that's what you're doing every day. So be careful to not fall into that trap.

Martha, friend number three, makes a few poor choices. She recently bought memberships to several online streaming sites to watch more of her favourite shows. She's also been trying out the recipes from the new dessert book she bought. Furthermore, she's

2   P Lally, C van Jaarsfeld, et al (2009) 'How are habits formed: Modelling habit formation in the real world', *European Journal of Social Psychology* Vol 40(6): 998.

decided to use the new coffee shop beside her work-place and add a chocolate macchiato to her lunch every day. Black coffee is boring, and she wants to spice it up a little. Nothing crazy, just a small change here and there.

At the end of six months, no perceivable difference exists among the three women.

Linda keeps doing what she's always done. Sarah continues to read a little bit every night and listen to audiobooks during her commute; Martha is 'enjoying' life and doing less. Even though each has their own pattern of behaviour, six months isn't long enough to see any real decline or improvement in their situations. True, Sarah may look a little leaner and Martha a little flabbier, but the changes are hardly noticeable.

Fast forward eighteen months:

Linda is in the same place as before.

Sarah looks leaner and is clearly more confident. She's read ten personal development books over the past eighteen months and has been using the tips to improve her quality of life.

Martha is very obviously putting on extra weight. Although she's caught up on her favourite TV shows, she hasn't progressed at work or in other areas of her life in the slightest.

At the end of twenty-five months, we start seeing measurable, visible differences in the women. At month twenty-seven, the difference is dramatic. By month thirty-one, the change is startling! Martha is now fat, while Sarah is trim. By simply cutting 125 calories a day, in thirty-one months Sarah has lost thirty-three pounds.

> 31 months = 940 days
> 940 days × 125 calories/day = 117, 500 calories
> 117,500 calories / 3,500 calories per pound =
> 33.5 pounds

Martha, who consumed 125 more calories a day during the same time period, gained 33.5 pounds. Now she weighs 67 pounds *more* than Sarah! But that's only the difference on the outside. It goes much deeper than that. Sarah invested almost one thousand hours in reading helpful books and listening to self-improvement audiobooks. Putting her newly gained knowledge into practice, she earned a promotion and a raise at work. Remember, if you want to earn more money, you need to deserve more money. Best of all, owing to the income and confidence she has gained, her marriage is thriving as well.

Martha, by contrast, is also unhappy at work. Thirty-one months have passed, she still holds the same position at work and her pay hasn't improved. Also, with the increased weight gain, she's unhappy with her body image and has started to project it onto the people closest to her. Her marriage is now on the rocks because of it.

Linda? Well, Linda is pretty much exactly where she was two and a half years ago, except more bitter about her situation as other people have improved their lives while she's still in the same place.

This is a fictitious story, of course, but it illustrates how making small and seemingly insignificant changes can lead to lasting results over time. It really is that simple.

But what if you're of an impatient constitution and want results faster? Easy: make more drastic changes. As long as what you're doing is sustainable and aligned with your specific goal, the rate or scale of the change you make is very much down to your personal preference and personality type. Just make sure that it is sustainable and that you stick to it. There's a reason you learn to walk before you can run. If you try and run before you walk, you are more likely to fall.

I spent years on autopilot like Linda, and nothing ever changed in my life. Several years ago, I decided to start getting up a little earlier than usual every day so that I wasn't rushing out the door stressed every morning. It started with just setting my alarm ten minutes earlier than usual, and instead of hitting snooze six times, I hit it five times. Over the next six months, I cut back each snooze alarm until I got down to just one snooze, and eventually I was able to get up as soon as the alarm went off.

Within a year, I was up a full hour before my previous wake-up time. With this extra time, I started to develop a morning routine around things that would improve my quality of life.

My muscular system has been always tight from years of training and playing sports. I hadn't been able to touch my toes since I was a kid, and I always complained that I just 'didn't have time' to stretch. As stretching is something I don't really enjoy doing, I can never find the motivation to do it after training or work, so I added it to my morning routine. Now I do it every day. My workouts are better – I don't feel as stiff and rigid I used to, and I can touch my toes for the first time in years! Now that it's a habit, I feel weird when I don't do it.

Another thing I started doing was listening to an audiobook or podcast during my morning routine. A few years ago, when I moved my fitness business online, I started working from an office in my house, so I wasn't getting to listen to audiobooks during my regular morning work commute anymore. Therefore, I paired audiobooks with my morning stretches – two birds with one stone.

Over the past three years, I have honed and continue to tweak this routine, and it works as my foundation pillar for the day. For years, I would rush out and start my day in a 'reactive' mode because I didn't give myself time in the morning. This compounded to more stress, more anxiety and a constant state of 'go, go, go'. Now the compound effect has worked in the opposite direction. My morning routine sets the pace and mood for my entire day and keeps me calmer, more productive and more creative as I'm not in a 'reactive' mode as soon as I wake up. The people who nurture their daily habits and use the positive nature of the compound effect appear to be an 'overnight success' or to have more than twenty-four hours in a day, but the truth is they've just learned to use the power of the compound effect. Once you understand the compound effect, the next step is making sure your fear doesn't stop you.

7

Rewire Fear – Feel the Fear and Do It Anyway

In *The Fitness Mindset*, I mentioned that my favourite acronym for fear is 'False Evidence Appearing Real', and the more I experience different challenges, the more this acronym proves true. Fear is natural, and we all feel it when we're moving towards a specific goal or faced with something unknown. Unfortunately, most people let fear stop them from taking the necessary steps to achieve what they truly want. I've learned over the years from working with, interviewing or associating with some incredible people that successful people feel the fear along with the rest of us, but they just don't let it stop them.

The week before I flew out to the Sahara to run six back-to-back marathons carrying all my food and supplies on my back, I had countless nightmares. I probably slept so well when I arrived in the desert because my previous nights were consumed by dreams of poisonous snakes (I was required to have a venom pump within arms' reach at all times) and getting lost in the middle of nowhere, followed by the thought that I'd dehydrate and die.

Again, this was all False Evidence Appearing Real, but try to tell my subconscious that at the time. I was freaking terrified! To give you a gauge of how scared I actually was, in this chapter I've included a note I wrote to myself the day before I flew out. One of the ways I deal with my own issues, insecurities or fears is writing out exactly what's going through my head at the time. I do this for two reasons:

The first reason is that it gets all those thoughts spiralling in my head out on paper and generally makes me feel less anxious about a given situation.

The second reason is probably more important. Writing serves as a reference point when dealing with future fears. I knew once I came out the other side of the particular fear (the Sahara, in this case) I was going to be able to reflect on that note the next time I was scared to do something new. It served as an anchor for the legs on my confidence table. If I'm feeling afraid before I step on stage to give a talk or have another potentially life-changing event, I go back and read how I felt in that moment, and all those fears tend to subside. Although my fears don't go away, they become manageable. Paralysing fear is generally replaced with cautious optimism, and the 'I can't do this' negative self-talk is replaced by, 'You felt this way before, and you did it then; you'll be fine'.

I'm aware I sound crazy in the note, but I've left the exact wording unedited and unaltered, so you can judge for yourself. A small exception is that, for the print version of the book, I have added asterisks into the swear words. Although I swear quite frequently in my everyday life, I dislike how it looks on the written page. But otherwise, the note is exactly as written on the original day. I should also mention that in the note I alternate between the first and third person, probably because of my panicked state of mind.

On the 'Rewire Your Mindset' section of my website, www.briankeanefitness.com, I've also added a video from one of my 'Rewire Your Mindset' seminars where I expand on what my feelings were when I wrote the note. In the video, I go through each line and explain my thought process at the time of writing.

Rereading the note below when I'm challenged with any new obstacle reinforces my belief that, although I'm always going to feel scared, I just need to feel the fear and do it anyway.

I'm feeling really scared today. The subconscious fear of the unknown is really playing on my mind today. Damn camel spiders the size of my head, poisonous snakes or those damn death scorpions – f*ck the f*cking desert!

Side note: Always check your shoes in the morning for scorpions. Now you're even worrying about stupid sh*t like your business, money, your investments, all projected fear elsewhere, this is clearly me subconscious trying to distract me as these aren't real problems, they're perceived problems. These distractions aren't helpful either, they're not even rational so be careful and catch them when they enter your mind, don't let them mindlessly intrude and create problems that aren't really there. You need to be mentally stronger, stop being a f*cking wimp and control that! They're your thoughts, control the f*cking things! Okay back to the fear Brian, focus. I know I'm going to finish [the six back-to-back marathons] and get over the finish line, even if I have to crawl. Motherf*cker, you will be carried out of there in a f*cking ambulance or you will cross that finish line. You've committed now shut the f*ck up and stop worrying. The work is done. Worrying is needlessly wasted energy now. Feel the fear, do it anyways. Think of mum, think of Holly (my daughter), but also think of the people who said that's you'd never survive this. Think about all those people that called you a loser. Think about all those people who doubted you. Use it all as fuel for the fire. Let your why drive you and use the negatively as power pillage. You think I can't do it? You just wait, and I'll f*cking show you that I can!!! Fear is false evidence appearing real.

As I said, I intentionally haven't edited the note as it gives you insights into exactly what was going through my head the day before I flew out. Any time you step into the unknown, you're going to come face to face with fears, and it's scary. But it's also relative. For you, it might be stepping into a gym for the first time; for someone else, it's approaching that person they're attracted to; and for others, it's asking for that raise or promotion at work. Your fear is relative, but the inoculation against it is the same for everyone – feeling it and doing it anyway. Behind every fear of yours is the person you want to be, and just because it's unknown doesn't mean that it's bad. As a matter of fact, nearly all the great things in life come on the other side of fear and struggle.

I spent far too much of my life choosing known hells in the place of unknown heavens. I would stay in jobs and relationships that made me miserable because they were 'what I knew', and I was afraid of change. I never challenged myself physically because of the fear of failure; I would stay in my comfort zone where I felt safe. This is still a daily battle because life is transient; it's always changing, and one needs to change with it. When I feel like not attacking something because I'm afraid of it, I often remind myself of a story I read once about a young man at the firing line.

The young man at the firing line

As the story goes, a young man had been captured behind enemy lines during a war and was sentenced to death by a firing squad. But the night before the execution was to take place, he was offered another option. Either he could face the firing squad the next morning, or he could walk out of the door at the back of the building. Upon learning his options, the man asked the captain, 'What is on the other side of that door?' 'No one knows', responded the captain, 'only unknown horrors'. The man pondered the choices throughout the night. The next morning, he chose the firing squad. After the shots rang out, the captain's secretary asked him what was beyond the door. The captain responded, 'Freedom. But very few people will select freedom because it is unknown.'

Although this story is extreme and probably apocryphal, it rings true in many of our lives. Some people will choose known hells over unknown heavens. This is how I lived for most of my early twenties. This is how many people live today. I see them. I've worked with them. I see them at the gym and sporting events. They are going through their own hell or unhappiness because deciding to make a change is too scary when the outcome of that change is unknown.

A lot of people never live their dream. Many never do the things they want to do. They stay in jobs that make them miserable. They stay in relationships that are destructive to their spirit. We put ourselves in self-imposed prisons and think we're stuck. You're not stuck; you are one decision away from changing your entire life. You are not a tree; if you don't like where you are, then move!

Just to clarify so that I'm not misunderstood, there are going to be times when life will knock you down and suffering is a part of growth, but that's not what I'm referring to here. Life has knocked me down several times. I am not asking you to run away from your problems. In fact, if you're feeling really brave, run towards them and see how quickly they fall when you start to attack them head on. If that's too much to ask, I am saying if you have tried to improve any given situation but to no avail, then it might be time to get your ladder against another wall.

If you are in a relationship where you have to constantly question the other person's trust or loyalty, it may be a sign that your ladder is against the wrong wall. If you are working a job that makes you miserable and ill when Monday morning rolls around, it's probably time to start moving your ladder. If your health is keeping you from doing the things you want to do in life, then it's time to make a change.

Change is never easy, and starting over is even harder. As Robin Sharma, the author of *The Monk Who Sold His Ferrari*, said, 'Change is difficult at the beginning, messy in the middle and beautiful at the end'.[1] When things are difficult at the start, just think about the compound effect and how much easier it will become when that inevitably kicks in. If you are not where you want to be, don't blame anyone else or your circumstances for it. Take responsibility for where you are and own the fact that you are the one choosing

---

[1]   R Sharma (1996) *The Monk Who Sold His Ferrari*. San Francisco: HarperCollins.

unhappiness over change. There's nothing wrong if that's what you've done up until now, but given that you're consciously aware of it, it's up to you to decide what you do next. Never forget that you're one decision away from changing any area of your life.

Every day is a new day – a new day to set new goals, a new day to take a different direction. No one on this earth is promised tomorrow, and, sadly, I can't guarantee a change in your life will make you happy, but I sure as hell can guarantee that if you are currently unhappy and don't make a conscious choice and effort to change, you will remain the same. If you don't change anything, nothing will change, and, as one my mentors used to say, 'If you keep doing what you're doing, you'll keep getting what you got'.

Why are we so fearful?

Millions of years ago, fear was our body's way of signalling that we were out of our comfort zone. It alerted us to possible dangers and gave us the burst of adrenaline we needed to run away. It's our basic flight-or-fight signal. Unfortunately, even though this response was useful in the days when a sabre-toothed tiger chased us, today most of the threats we face are not all that life threatening. They're mostly perceived threats. We worry about our job security, our social status, or the opinions of others about what we do or say. In some cases, we even catastrophise a situation and start making up stories about all the things that can possibly go wrong. Again, it is an example of your own worst enemy living between your two ears.

I remember attending a party when I was about twenty-one. The party was mostly attended by people I wasn't very familiar with, and I only knew one person there. I've always had to deal with the social anxiety that comes from being in large groups. The anxiety I felt was crippling as a teenager, and it's something I still have to manage to this day. I still have to lean into that discomfort every time I'm in a big crowd as I'm hardwired to want to run away from it.

Given that, alcohol – being the great social lubricant that it is – helped me a lot throughout much of my earlier life. The only reason I attended the party was that I knew a young woman I liked was also attending and I really wanted to talk to her. The entire night, I was preoccupied with approaching her and introducing myself properly.

Several drinks into the night, I finally got my chance, and, with all the courage four beers can give, I approached her. We talked for about twenty minutes and actually got along really well. I made her laugh a few times, after which I asked her for her number. To my delight – and astonishment – she gave it to me.

Being the awkward young guy who felt the need to fill any silence in a conversation, I made some silly joke about calling her. I can't even remember the exact line, but it was something like 'Here's my number for a 3am call' or something stupid like that. My attempt at being funny was met with an unimpressed facial expression.

Picking up on the cue, I awkwardly changed the subject. We talked for another ten minutes, and then she had to leave. Success, right? Before the night had started, I had planned to talk to this woman and would have given my right arm to get her phone number. Surely, this was better than I ever expected, and I should be ecstatic. Not quite.

The encounter, thirty minutes of good conversation, the exchange of phone numbers and even a warm embrace upon leaving, but do you think that's what my mind focused on? Nope. It focused on the silly comment I made and her reaction. When something good happens to you, you initially feel great. Then, suddenly, your mind is hijacked, and you start to focus on the one thing that went wrong. If you have ever done this, then you know exactly what happened next.

My negative self-talk started to kick in: 'You idiot, Brian, why did you say that? You're such a fool. I bet this isn't even her real phone number!' and similar unsupportive thoughts raced through my mind. So often we let our minds be hijacked by such thoughts; we focus on the one negative thing and forget about all the positives. Such tendencies can be crippling for your self-confidence.

I never did call that woman, and this was one of the many times over the following years when I let false evidence become real and let my biggest enemy live between my two ears. Before he died, my granddad told me, 'You never regret the mistakes you make or the chances you took [your failure always serves as feedback], but when you look back on your life, you only regret the chances you didn't take'. I never forgot those words.

The mind is hardwired through evolution to focus on the negative things. If you heard a rustle in the bushes, it was better to think the worst and run away in case it was a sabre-toothed tiger or something higher on the food chain. If you assumed it was a gust of wind, then you ended up somebody else's lunch. This hardwiring has been passed down from generation to generation. The hunter-gatherers who fled and survived successfully passed on their genes to us. They're our ancestors. You can thank them for that, but don't forget that what kept them alive thousands of years ago only serves to make you miserable today.

Behind every fear is a person you want to be

Some people will do anything to avoid the uncomfortable feeling of fear. If you are one of those people, you run an even bigger risk of never getting what you want in any of the four quadrants. Remember, following the path of least resistance is for electricity, not for you. When you do what is easy, your life will be hard, but when you make a conscious choice to do what is hard, in most cases your life will become easier. Most good things in life require taking a risk, especially calculated risks where you weigh the upsides and downsides and ask yourself if you can handle the downsides. Still, the nature of risk is that it doesn't always work out. People do lose their investments; people do forget their words during public speeches; people do die in the Sahara. But as the adage goes, 'Nothing ventured, nothing gained'.

How to get rid of fear?

'I have lived a long life and had many troubles, most of which never happened.'
— Mark Twain

There are a few strategies you can use to get rid of fear. The ones that work for you are subjective to your personality type, so I advise experimenting with them all and doubling down on the ones that work best for you.

I. Imagine the worst-case scenario

Have you ever worried about something only for it to happen and not be as bad as you thought? One way to make your fear disappear is to ask yourself, 'Is what I'm imagining the worst-case scenario?' If it is, great, then play out the scenario from the start to the end like a movie. If the version playing in your head isn't the worst-case scenario, for the purpose of this strategy, alter it until it is.

At the time I was planning to leave my full-time teaching job to start my business, I was terrified of making the switch. I had spent years climbing the ladder against that particular wall, securing degrees and jobs to ascend that hierarchical structure. I was wrapped up in a story that was a combination of the sunk cost fallacy – 'Have I wasted all these years?' – and the fear of the lack of a regular pay cheque after having been conditioned to receive one for years.

It took me nearly two years to make the decision to leave the teaching job, but the moment of clarity came when I had been sitting down with my mum at Christmas. I had told her my fears about wasting all that time and money only to quit now. I also expressed my fears of not having a steady pay cheque to rely on. Then, she asked me, 'Okay, so what if it all fails? Your new business doesn't work out, you go broke… What do you do then?' I replied, 'I'd have to go back to teaching full time'. To my shock and surprise, she asked, 'So you're telling me you'd be in exactly the same situation as you are in now?' I handed in my resignation letter the following week.

Playing out your worst-case scenario can be an effective measure in helping you deal with the things you fear. Generally, it's never as bad as you think.

Alternatively, you can dramatise the worst-case scenario until it gets so ridiculous that you either laugh it off or all sting has been removed from it. For example, sticking with my above scenario, let's say starting my business didn't work out and, for some strange reason, teaching was no longer a viable option. Maybe my degree certificate got blown away in a storm; maybe the university lost all my student records. (As it happens in this fictitious worst-case scenario, the week before a virus attack had resulted in the deletion of the records of every 'Brian Keane' who had graduated from all the databases at my uni. Just bad timing, I guess.) Also, my family and friends disowned me because of the embarrassment of being associated with somebody who tried to set up their own business and failed. Moreover, owing to the financial losses, I must live the rest of my life on the street, sharing my new cardboard-box home with a pet raccoon. At least I have pet raccoon! I named him Jamie. There's always a silver lining.

Obviously, this is a ridiculous scenario, but it really does take the sting off the situation. If you really want to have fun with it, share the issue you're pondering with one of your best friends and give brownie points for the most ridiculous inclusions in the scenario. I've done this with my inner circle, and it has amazed me how some people excel with a good problem, a bottle of tequila and an unfiltered conversation!

Of course, sometimes the risks are real. My worst-case scenario of running the marathons through the Sahara was I would be bitten by a poisonous snake and die, but I made a calculated risk. I kept my venom pump within arms' reach at all times, I stayed hydrated and fuelled myself as best as I could, and I checked the GPS regularly to make sure I was always in reach of rescue if needed. That's an extreme example, and I don't recommend taking such big risks casually. But lying on my deathbed in seventy years, I would have regretted not doing it out of fear. I went through the worst-case scenario, then calculated and minimised the risks. I felt the fear and did it anyway, and I've never regretted it.

2. Anchor a time when you triumphed in the face of fear

Have you ever jumped off a diving board? If so, you probably remember the first time you walked to the edge of the board and looked down. The water looked a lot deeper than it really was. Considering the distance from the board and your eyes to the water, it probably looked like a very long way down, too.

You were scared. If you were scared of heights, you were maybe even terrified. But did you look at your mum or dad or diving instructor and say, 'You know, I'm just afraid to do this right now. I think I'll go do some therapy on this, and if I get rid of my fear, I'll come back and try again… '?

Hell no, you didn't say that!

You felt the fear, somehow mustered the courage and jumped into the water. You felt the fear and did it anyway. When you brought your head to the surface again, you probably swam with all you had to the edge of the pool, thankful for something to grab onto, with a rush of adrenaline, probably feeling a mild rush of ecstasy. More than likely, you also felt a wave of achievement wash over you. I'll even go as far to bet that after a minute or two, you went up and did it again and again and again, enough times that it started to get really fun.

Such experiences add one more leg to your confidence table. You knew you had to do something, and even though everything inside you screamed not to, you did it anyway. Experiences like this don't have to come from diving off a high board. Once upon a time, taking a college or intra-level job exam or learning to drive were terrifying experiences, but somehow you figured them out. Your first kiss was another terrifying experience at one stage in your life, but now it's unlikely to cause you any distress.

Difficult situations normalise with experience; the fear sting is removed with experience. That's how everything is when it comes to fear! Every time you expose yourself to the thing you're afraid of, its power over you gradually reduces. The next time you feel like approaching someone at a bar or asking your boss for a raise, remember the other times when you were afraid and anchor them in your mind when working towards future goals.

That's another reason why fitness and exercise can be so powerful. If you're someone who can't run more than a mile at a time, set yourself the goal to run 3 miles. Once you do it, your confidence will grow. If you could barely move the barbell the first time you did a bench press or squat but now you regularly add a couple of plates either side, that's another example of using the other areas in your life to grow your confidence. Use your previous success as anchors for future goals.

The first time I ever stepped on a bodybuilding stage, I was petrified. I had grown up idolising people like Arnold Schwarzenegger and always dreamt of doing a bodybuilding show some day. The night before my first event, I trembled with anxiety, worried about falling over on stage, forgetting my poses or, worse, being laughed at for being too small. All I wanted out of that show was to not be humiliated. To my surprise, I actually finished in the top four out of twenty-seven other competitors. It wasn't so much the finish that left an impression on me but the memory of how I felt the night before. For the first time in my entire life, I walked towards the fear instead of running away. This experience served as a reference point for a lot of my future subjective successes in the other areas of my life. I had added one giant leg to my confidence table.

Stepping on stage in bodybuilding shows and running six back-to-back marathons couldn't be further from one other in the world of fitness, but for me the unease they brought were comparable. Every time I would get caught up in negative self-talk – 'I wasn't a runner' or 'I was not going to be able to run through the Sahara' – I would go back to the night before my first bodybuilding show and use that as a success anchor to get me to the finish line in the Sahara. When I ran through the Arctic Circle in February 2019, I did exactly the same. The fear never goes away; you just get better at handling it. Every time I worried about the 230km distance or the -38°C temperature in the Arctic, I reminded myself that I once thought running six back-to-back marathons in the Sahara was impossible. Nothing is impossible. If somebody else has done it, they're living proof that it can be done. Redefine your impossible if you have to.

3. Distraction techniques

The last strategy is a little bit of a short-term one, but it can work tremendously well if you have fully committed to the end goal – such as joining the gym or asking for a raise at work or running a 3-mile race – beforehand. It's worth noting that this technique is one of the worst things you can do if you haven't fully committed yet as it can actually take you backwards by shifting your eyes off the figurative ball.

Short bursts of distraction can get you out of your own head, especially when you're fully committed to attacking something you are clearly afraid of. If you've signed up to give a speech or go to the gym for the first time, identify the times you feel most anxious or scared. For most people, the intensity of the feeling increases the closer they are to the event. Therefore, have your pre-planned distractions ready to go.

Your distraction may be reading a fiction book series that immerses you, watching movies of a genre you love or spending time with your loved ones. It doesn't really matter what it is. As long as it makes you forget about the thing you're afraid of, it can work very effectively. It's also worth considering that every minute you spend worrying about it is needless suffering. Seneca said, 'A man who suffers before it is necessary, suffers more than is necessary', which basically means overthinking a situation leads you to suffer twice – once before it happens and again during the event.[2] You will generally find that the event is not as bad as you thought. Obviously, in the case of running through the Sahara, that wasn't true – it hurt like hell. But, in most cases, thinking about the event is normally worse than the actual event.

The week before running through the Sahara, I went through more movies and fiction books than I had in the previous six months combined! As my anxiety and fear tend to peak before I go to bed, I consciously set aside some distraction time for those anxious hours so that they didn't negatively affect my sleep. Meditating, exercising and listening to music are all great options, too, so find what works best for you and use that as your strategic distraction.

4. Be willing to pay the price

I greatly appreciate the quote 'If people knew how hard I had to work to gain my mastery, it wouldn't seem so wonderful at all' that is often attributed to the great artist Michelangelo. This goes for nearly anything

---

2   From the book *Letters From a Stoic* by Seneca the Younger, published in 65 AD.

that's worth having. A person who is in great shape has created the right habits around food choices, has consistently built training into their life schedule and does it consistently to reap the benefits of the compound effect.

The people in incredible relationships don't just show up with flowers on Valentine's Day and ignore their partner for the rest of the year. They do the right things every day that strengthen the relationship – listening to one another, building the trust in each other and working through problems instead of burying their heads in the sand and avoiding them.

Successful entrepreneurs or business owners didn't just wake up with a fortune in their bank accounts. They found a way to provide a service or product that helps people or upskilled their knowledge until companies or corporations were willing to pay them extraordinary amounts of money for their expertise and knowledge.

Behind every great achievement is a story of education, training, practice, discipline and sacrifice. If you want the gold at the end of the rainbow, you have to be willing to pay the price. Beware that the price may be pursuing one activity while putting everything else in your life on hold. I did this in 2015 when I finished eighth in the Fitness Model World Championships. Although a micro imbalance can lead to a macro balance over the long term, in this case, that was not what happened, and the other areas of my life suffered.

Therefore, it's important to recognise when it's worth paying the price and when it's not.

As I mentioned earlier, one of the reasons I created the four quadrants was to avoid such imbalances ever happening again. However, if that 'all in' or 'complete focus on one goal' approach is still a tool in your toolkit, be careful that it doesn't become your only strategy. Going 'all in' towards a target may be the price you have to pay for what you want right now, but be mindful that achieving your goal doesn't come at the expense of other equally important things.

While you're weighing up the price is normally a good time to take the 30,000-foot bird's eye view we talked about earlier so that other parts of your life don't collapse as you move towards your goal. A friend of mine once told me to 'never forget the flowers at one's feet when reaching for the moon', meaning not to forget the beautiful or amazing things that you have as you strive for what you want.

Flowers take years to grow but seconds to be destroyed. At the end of the day, awards, best-selling books and successful businesses mean nothing to me if my mum, daughter or inner circle don't respect me – or, even worse, hate me. Such a wide-angled view helps me when making decisions. Some of the things you want to do at the moment may require more time, effort and focus right now, and that's fine; just don't allow yourself to rocket to the moon only to realise you've crushed all the flowers that were once at your feet.

Being willing to pay the price may involve investing all of your wealth or savings. I went broke thrice trying to get my business off the ground. The last time was one of the lowest points in my life. I literally had to reach down and search the back of my couch to find money for a bus ride. I needed that money to get to my bank to take out a loan to pay my rent for that month. That was a low point, and I don't advise being in such a situation, as I made some pretty stupid financial decisions that could have easily been avoided if I had read the right books or contacted the right business consultants beforehand.

Nonetheless, as with all failure, those decisions gave me valuable feedback and served as the spark for acquiring the knowledge to make better investments in the future. They also allowed me to become more regimented with finances over the past several years. This change has led to more than several prosperous investments and is another example of how a seed of failure can bear a fruit of success. Failure really is the gift that keeps on giving if you choose to learn from it.

Normally, a price people have to pay to find success is the willingness to walk away from the safety of a current situation. I spoke earlier about the fear of leaving unknown heavens for known hells, but this willingness may be much more subtle and dangerous. I call it the 'good is the death of great' or the 'yeah, it's okay' syndrome.

'Yeah, it's okay' syndrome

When I was working full time as a teacher, although there were times I hated the long hours marking books and attending needless meetings, I genuinely enjoyed the teaching and working directly with children.

In *The Fitness Mindset*, I mentioned that we tend to move away from pain and towards pleasure in nearly everything we do. This tendency makes a lot of decisions very easy to make as pain serves as an intensive driver for change. For example, if you feel much pain from the insecurity that comes from being 100 pounds overweight or not fitting into your favourite pair of jeans anymore, that can force you to change. Similarly, you feel so miserable and insecure in a relationship that it energises you to leave, or you hate your job so much that you use that emotion to gather the courage to quit.

It's significantly more difficult to make a change when things are 'okay'. If someone asks you about your job or your relationship and you reply, 'Yeah, it's okay', that may be a real cause for concern.

If you're reading this book, you're already an outlier in your thinking and there's a good chance you're not settling for average like other people you may know. But have you a blind spot somewhere? I spoke earlier about bridging the gap between the things you know, the things you don't know and the things you don't know you don't know. The parts of your life that are 'okay' can be the things you don't even know you don't know about. I inoculate against this syndrome by regularly asking myself in any given situation: 'If this was the only thing I get or have or do for the rest of life, would I be happy?'

For example, if this was the only romantic relationship I ever had, would I be happy (and is my ladder up against the right wall)? Or, if this was the only job I ever had, would I be happy to work here for the rest of my life (and is my ladder up against the right wall)?

When the answer is 'yes' more often than not, you know your ladder is against the right wall. If the answer is 'no', then it may be time to question whether your actions are mapping onto your ambition. I'll speak about the importance of goal setting in Chapter Eleven, and it's not the generic 'set a goal, work towards it, achieve it' strategy that you read in most goal-setting books; it goes into more specific details about what you need to do, who you need to become and how to set up the vision. For now, though, I want to highlight an idea from that chapter: *You need to know what the end goal is*.

You can't hit a target you cannot see, and if you just mindlessly continue doing what you're doing, you'll keep getting what you have. To get something new, you need to take different action steps, but none of that matters if you don't know what you want.

Ask yourself, 'What do I want? What kind I relationship do I want to be in? What kind of body do I want? What kind of job would I love?' Now ask yourself whether what you're currently doing is moving you closer or further away from those things. If it's moving you closer, keep going. Your ladder is against the right wall, so continue to climb. But if it's not, you need to change it.

It's a very simple question and an even simpler concept, but the answer can be earth-shattering if it's the first time you've asked it. As I told you earlier, that's what happened to me as I walked down the streets of East London, playing out my funeral in my mind.

Teaching was a job I liked, but I didn't love it. It was 'okay' and not bad enough to make a change but not good enough to feel fulfilled. Good or good enough really is the death of the great. Ask yourself whether you'd be happy if this job, relationship, diet or training programme were the only one you got for the rest of your life. Just be prepared for the answer that follows. If it's a painful answer, know that the pain is temporary.

Pain is temporary

Many things are typically required to reach a successful outcome. The willingness to do what's required adds an extra dimension to the mix and can help you persevere in the face of overwhelming challenges, setbacks, hardships, physical pain and even personal injuries.

I still remember the pain that coursed through my body while running my fourth marathon through the Sahara; it was like nothing I had ever experienced at the time. The fourth day was actually a double marathon – I had to cover 53.2 miles of sand dunes in less than forty-eight hours. It meant running through the Sahara in the middle of the night at -2°C temperature.

As I had spent the entire day running in 40°C weather, I was sweating profusely by the time night fell. As the temperature dropped, my bones began to hurt. My feet had been blistered from the previous three days of marathons, and I was hurting a lot.

After over twenty-one hours of running, I started to hallucinate. I saw shadows of people and snakes out of the corners of my eyes. I constantly tried to bring my focus back to the six inches in front of my face. Everything hurt. At times, I questioned whether I was going to be able to finish. The worst-case scenario of falling over and being eaten by a camel circulated in my mind (yes, I was severely dehydrated and genuinely thought I might be eaten by a camel).

I tried to not concentrate on the pain, but it kept creeping back in. I struggled but continued to put one foot in front of the other, step by step and mile by mile until I got to the finish line. Every step shot pain through me like the stab of a knife, and it hurt for weeks after. The blisters on my feet took about a month to heal. But pain is a funny thing – it doesn't last forever. With the exception of chronic pain, it's temporary.

The only thing that got me through the night was repeatedly telling myself, 'Pain is temporary; pain is temporary'. Although I knew the pain would go away, my mind was starting to rationalise quitting: 'Go on, quit! You've come far enough. You're not a runner anyway. Just blow the rescue whistle, click the GPS, do it, do it, do it.'

I knew if I clicked the GPS, a helicopter would

arrive within thirty minutes and swoop me out of the desert. I also knew that true character is tested under pressure, and if I quit, that would stay with me forever. I knew if I quit, a day would come when I would have to look my daughter in the eye and tell her I wasn't good enough and her dad was a loser. Although it may sound harsh, quitting because I was in pain would have made me a loser in my eyes.

Before I continue, I just want to clarify that losing and being beaten are not the same thing. Losing is when you make a conscious choice to give up because the task at hand is 'too difficult'. Being beaten is some-thing else. It means you've given everything you had, but the other person, place or thing was better on that given day or at that particular time. Losing and being beaten are not the same – never confuse the two.

There's nothing wrong with being beaten or even consciously deciding to stop something because you no longer feel the cost is worth the effort. If you did everything you could have – all the work, all the reps, all the sets, all the meetings – but you were still beaten or you consciously decided that it wasn't what you wanted anymore, then you're still a winner in my eyes. Just don't confuse the two and make up a story to justify quitting by telling yourself the task at hand is too difficult.

Quitting because the task at hand is 'too difficult' or because you can't handle the pain of striving to complete it is losing. Losing is a choice. That night, I made the choice that I wasn't telling my daughter her daddy was a loser. If something unforeseen hit me in the desert and I was beaten by the elements – trapped in a sandstorm, bitten by a snake, etc – the case would have been different. I wasn't going to put my life in jeopardy, but quitting because of the pain would have been losing.

As I said earlier, there's nothing wrong with changing direction, and you should always give yourself permission to change your mind on anything you do. By contrast, making the conscious choice to quit because of the pain, despite knowing your ladder is against the right wall, makes you a loser.

In the past, I quit runs because my legs were sore. I quit courses because they were 'too hard'. Hell, before the age of twenty-four, I quit nearly everything I ever signed up for! Then I realised physical, mental and even emotional pain, in most cases, go away. But quitting and knowing you gave up because you told yourself the task at hand was too difficult will stay with you forever.

To make a change in this regard, I had to own the fact that I had a weak mindset. It wasn't until I got real with myself and stopped making excuses and concocting stories about why I quit things that I was able to move forward and hit the targets I set for myself. Once you own that, previous losses become the fuel for the fire on your next venture. Every run I ever quit fuelled my ultramarathons. At mile 35 in a 52-mile race, I remembered what it felt like to quit. Somehow, it fuelled me to take one more step and then one more, and so on.

Every course I ever quit fuelled me to get my honours degrees in business, my postgraduate degree in teaching and all my certifications in sports nutrition, fitness and health. The days when I didn't want to study or the occasions when I couldn't concentrate because I was up all night caring for my sick daughter, I reminded myself how bad I felt when I quit. That served as the inspiration to set my alarm the next day and get my study hours in.

Nothing can change until you take responsibility for it. We all fail sometimes, and we all have quit something at some stage in our lives – a job, a workout programme or a relationship, among others. It's not about what you've done in the past, it's about asking yourself the question, 'What am I going to do about it *today*? What's Important Now (WIN)? Am I going to wallow in self-pity and blame the world for all my problems, or am I going to own my weaknesses and go get what I want?' My life didn't change until I realised that the choice was mine to make. Now ask yourself: 'What choice am I going to make?'

Never forget that the pain will go away and it's temporary. It may last for a day, a week, a month or even a year, but eventually it will subside. Quitting, on the other hand, lasts forever!

Also remember that it's all right to give something your all and be beaten or to even decide that the effort isn't worth it anymore and refocus your energy on something else. But losing, that's a choice.

8

Rewire Self-Discipline – You're Not Born with It; You Build It!

*'Perhaps the most valuable result of all education is
the ability to make yourself do the thing you have to do,
when it ought to be done, whether you like it or not.'*
— Thomas Henry Huxley

The golden thread of a highly successful and meaningful life is self-discipline. Discipline allows you to do all the things you know in your heart you should do but never feel like doing. Similar to the Thomas Huxley quote above, one of my mentors used to tell me that, 'Successful people do what they need to do whether they feel like it or not'. When I adopted this philosophy in my own life, my entire world changed.

The biggest misconception we hold is that people are born with self-discipline. For years, I would tell myself the story that the people who had the dedication to train for a marathon or bodybuilding show or those with the discipline to get up early were just born like that. They came into this world with something I didn't have. I would use the excuse that they had good genetics for running or bodybuilding and those early risers were probably morning people anyway and find it easy to get up at 5am.

Here's the truth: Nobody finds it easy to get up before sunrise. Every person you know who gets up early has trained themselves to do it. In my mid-twenties, I was fortunate to have had a brief encounter with a monk who gave me a great piece of advice on early rising: 'The only battle you should win every day is with the sun', meaning one should be up before the sun every day. As a 'five alarmer' – the term I use to describe people who set five alarms so that they can hit snooze several times before getting up (don't act like you've never done it) – I instantly recognised the concept of how beating the sun every day was valuable. Still, I didn't apply his advice at the time, and it took me another year before I adopted it. This was a case of knowing and not doing, which can be a breeding ground for mediocrity if repeated consistently over time.

I spent years trying to iron out the character flaw of 'knowing and not doing', and thankfully, like everything, it got easier over time. When you get into the habit of applying useful advice you've been given or, at the very least, experimenting, testing or trialling it for yourself, you start to realise that it was just fear or some story you told yourself that prevented you from making the change.

For example, my internal dialogue for not getting

up early went something like this: 'If I get up at 5am or 6am, I'll be tired. If I'm tired, I'll be grumpy at work, and my work colleagues won't like me. Also, if I'm tired, I'll skip the gym, and then I'll feel even worse. No, I'll just stick with getting up at 7.30am. That's what I know, and that's what I'm comfortable with.'

Once you question such stories and realise they're just opinions or fear disguised as practicality, you can start to change them. Oftentimes, it's just having to step outside of your comfort zone, and although this is hard at first, getting comfortable being uncomfortable can be learned.

Regarding getting up early, I knew what I had to do, but I still didn't do it. Soon, I would realise that every scenario where I knew what I had to do but still didn't do it came down to a lack of self-discipline. When I mindlessly ate sugar-, fat- and salt-laden foods that weren't factored into my nutritional plan, it was due to a lack of self-discipline. When I skipped the gym because I was tired after work, it was because of a lack of self-discipline. Even when I procrastinated on work tasks, it was down to a lack of self-discipline. When I started to treat self-discipline like a muscle that needed to be built and strengthened, everything started to change.

Self-discipline, like so many other things I suggest doing in this book, is a choice. You build it and make it stronger; you're not born with it! I spent most of my early adult life admiring other people who did things I dreamt of doing, but I never believed I could be the same as them. Even on the days I felt more confident about my abilities, I had no blueprint for how to do what they did and would just give up after a few minutes of convincing myself that it was too hard and wasn't worth the time or effort. I eventually got around this tendency by realising that anything truly worth having is nearly always hard to get.

People often ask me how I can be so passionate when I speak. I'm passionate when I speak because it is their lives I'm talking about. When I'm telling you to set goals, create the right habits and get your ladder up against the right wall, I'm not telling you all that to sell more books. Hell, read this book and give it to your friend for free when you're done. I'm writing these words because I'm talking about your life!

True, it's great to know how well your favourite sports team is doing in the league or which celebrity is dating whom, and yes, you should factor in some form of escapism or disconnection from your day. But, if you know more about your favourite sports team or celebrity than about who you are or what makes you happy, and you're complaining you don't have what you want, then your priorities are all messed up.

I spent years learning every stat of every player of my favourite sports team, and I could tell you which celebrity was cheating on whom, but I couldn't tell you what I wanted or the things that made me happy. It was too difficult to ask those questions and even harder to apply the answers. But like everything, you get to a 'fed-up' point and hit your figurative wall of pain when something needs fixing. I realised I was living a life of dying at twenty-five but not being buried until I was eighty, and something had to change.

Once you make the decision to make a change, you need to build one personality trait – self-discipline – and everything else will fall into place. As the saying goes, 'Nothing works until you do the work.' As important as it is to have an end vision of what you want to achieve, until you build the self-discipline to do what you need to do whether you want to or not, your final jigsaw piece will always be missing.

As I said above, the beauty of self-discipline is that it's like a muscle; the more you work it, the stronger it becomes. The stronger it gets, the more habitual using it becomes, and the compound effect kicks in.

I have three pillars of self-discipline that I regularly come back to every day. Every strong house has a solid foundation, and these pillars operate as my foundation for self-discipline and mental toughness. Your pillars may be different, and I advise you to experiment with a few different things that you know make you mentally stronger and help you get closer to your end goal. My end goal is to make sure the world is a little bit better because I have been here as well as grow and feed the relationships with the people who will cry when I die. Although your goals may be completely different, these pillars can serve as a foundation for anything you hope to achieve moving forward.

I. Getting up early

The reason getting up early works so well as a foundation pillar of self-discipline is that it literally comes at the start of your day. I can't speak for everyone, and I know some people enjoy mornings more than others, but I *hate* mornings. My body never wants to get up on the first alarm, and it still takes me twenty minutes to remember my name every single morning. As I mentioned earlier, I used to set five alarms so that I could hit snooze four times before I actually had to get up. Still, along with following the next pillar, my entire life started to change in 2015 when I joined the 5am club. The 5am club is just what I call people who regularly rise before the sun every day.

When I started making the change, as I was used to getting up at 7.30am I set the target small at first. To start with, I decided to give myself an extra hour in the morning to build a morning routine, so I started setting my alarm ten minutes earlier every week until I was getting up at 6.30am. Six weeks later, I adjusted my target from 6am to 5.30am and onward until I finally reached 5am.

Now you may think, 'There's no way I'm getting up at 5am', and that was what I thought at the beginning, too. Just start with setting the alarm ten to twenty minutes before you normally get up. I advise using this time to collect your thoughts, do some exercise or just think about your day. After a few weeks, it will become ingrained as a habit, and you can decide if you want to keep shifting the time until you get to the 5am club. That hour or two between 5am and 7am, before the whole world wakes up, can be incredible at reducing your stress or anxiety levels.

I never made the connection between my habit of jumping out of bed on the fifth alarm, rushing through breakfast and running out the door, and my high levels of anxiety and stress throughout the day. If you start your day in a highly reactive state, that's how your entire day is going to go. If you own your morning, you can own your day.

2. Read every day

When I am asked at seminars how I went from working as a financially struggling teacher in London to building an incredibly successful online fitness business, my answer is always the same. It came from the combination of getting up earlier and reading more. As I've mentioned throughout this book, you need to learn from mistakes, but nobody said they have to be your mistakes.

Books are probably the single best way to fill in those gaps between what you don't know and what you don't know you don't know. The billionaire investor Charlie Munger asks us to 'make friends with the imminent dead', meaning learn from the greats who have gone before you.[1] Some of your favourite authors

---

[1]   C Munger and P D Kaufman (2005) *Poor Charlie's Almanack*. Missouri: Walsworth Publishing Company.

may still be alive; most of mine are, and it's vital to use their stories, advice or tips to enhance and move your life forward.

I like to think of reading books as mining for gold; you're just looking for one nugget of gold in every book you read. If you read twelve books a year (one per month), you gain twelve nuggets of gold that can potentially move your life forward in some meaningful way if you apply the knowledge learned. That works out as 120 books over 10 years! Now let the compound effect kick in and see how quickly your life changes.

Some books will give you significantly more than one nugget of gold. I even hope that this book serves as one of those for you as my personal favourites teach me a lesson nearly every time I read them. The pre-Socratic Greek philosopher Heraclitus is said to have observed that a person 'cannot go into the same river twice', meaning that the person and the river are different every time.[2] New water has flowed into the river, and new experiences or knowledge have flowed into the person. That's the exact reason why I reread my favourite books every year. Every time I reread a book, my life is generally in a different place, so the message I get from the book is different every time. When and if you read this book a second (or third or fourth) time, different sections will likely jump out at you as your

---

2 See the 'I never understood Heraclitus' river analogy...'
   Q&A post on the Ask Philosophers website (15 Oct. 2005).
   www.askphilosophers.org/question/202, accessed 2 Oct. 2019.

priorities will have changed since you read it the first time. Like the river in the quote above, great books are a little different every time you read them.

Some of my favourite books, in no particular order, are:

- *Poor Charlie's Almanack* by Charlie Munger, compiled by Peter D Kaufman[3]
- *The Monk Who Sold His Ferrari* by Robin Sharma[4]
- *Letters from a Stoic* by Seneca[5]
- *Thinking, Fast and Slow* by Daniel Kahneman[6]
- *Mastery* by Robert Greene[7]
- *Meditations* by Marcus Aurelius[8]
- *12 Rules for Life* by Jordan Peterson[9]
- *The Obstacle Is the Way* by Ryan Holiday[10]

I have other favourites too, and I regularly update them on my blog at www.briankeanefitness.com, but all those mentioned above have permanent positions on my bookshelf.

Until the age of twenty-four, I had read a total of maybe four non-academic books, and they were mainly

---

3   C Munger and P D Kaufman (2005) *Poor Charlie's Almanack*. Missouri: Walsworth Publishing Company.
4   Robin Sharma (1996) *The Monk Who Sold His Ferrari*. San Francisco: HarperCollins.
5   *Letters from a Stoic* by Seneca published in 65 AD.
6   D Kahneman (2011) *Thinking, Fast and Slow*. New York: Farrar, Straus and Giroux.
7   R Greene (2012) *Mastery*. New York: Viking Adult.
8   *Meditations* by Marcus Aurelius 161–180 AD. First translation in 1792 by Richard Graves.
9   J Peterson (2018) *12 Rules for Life*. Canada: Penguin Random House.
10   R Holiday (2014) *The Obstacle is the Way*. New York: Penguin.

sports autobiographies. When I made the conscious decision to read more (mostly audiobooks at first), I started to see things move forward in all the four quadrants of my life in a positive direction. If this is the first book you have ever read, great, use it as a springboard for others. Remember the Chinese proverb, 'The best time to plant a tree was twenty years ago; the next best time is today'.

3. Work out regularly

I'm going to approach the foundation pillar of working out regularly from a slightly different angle. As someone with a fitness and sports background, it's easy to get labelled as one of those people who finds exercise easy or, at the very least, enjoys it. I concur that label is correct to a degree. I enjoy most physical exercises, especially weightlifting and high-intensity training. I even like swimming and cycling, but there's one form of exercise that I truly hate – running. Yes, the person who has run multiple marathons through the Sahara and the Arctic Circle hates to run! But that's exactly why I do it.

I joke with my ultramarathon friends (who love to run) that I hate every single step of running from when I step out the front door or onto the treadmill until I'm back home or off the treadmill. I find it so difficult. But every single time I do it, it makes me mentally stronger.

Nearly every training day, I run for this reason. The tougher you are on yourself, the easier life will be on you. As I trained myself to lean into the discomfort every day, the impact extends to other parts of my life. You get comfortable being unconformable, so when you are forced to have a conversation you really don't want to have with a loved one or co-worker, you just do it anyway.

When you're tired at the end of a workday and just want to watch TV instead of playing with or reading to your kids, you get off the couch and make a jigsaw puzzle or read a story to them. Self-discipline is like a muscle, and you make it stronger by exercising it. Every morning I get up early and run, the two things that contribute to a better version of myself and make the whole day feel easier. Day by day, you build that muscle of doing what you need to do whether you feel like it or not.

The quality of your life is ultimately determined by the quality of your choices and decisions – the career choices you make, the books you read, the time you wake up every morning and the thoughts you have during the day. Your foundation pillars may not be to get up early every day or run. One of your pillars may be to not let people walk all over you anymore or start making your lunch the night before so that you make better food choices the following day; it may even be to finally stick to a gym programme after all these years. Regardless of what it is, as long as it's challenging you it's building that discipline.

When you consistently flex your willpower by making the choices you know are the right ones (rather than the easy ones), you take back control of your entire life. I've learned from mentors, books and experiences that effective, fulfilled people do not spend their time doing what is most convenient and comfortable. They have the courage to listen to their own voice but ignore it when it's not helping. They do what they have to do, as opposed to what they want to do. It's this habit that makes them great.

Aristotle said it better than I ever could:

> Whatever we learn to do, we learn by actually doing it. Men come to be builders, for instance, by building, and harp players, by playing the harp. The same way, by doing just acts, we come to be just; by doing self-controlled acts, we come to be self-controlled; and by doing brave acts, we come to be brave.[II]

If you want to be more self-disciplined, practice self-discipline and do it every day until it becomes a habit. Once the compound effect kicks in, the changes that result are like magic to people looking in from the outside. Self-discipline just becomes a habit.

II   R Holiday (2016) *The Daily Stoic*. London: Profile Books.

9

Rewire Your Habits

Some psychologists believe that up to 90% of our behaviours are habitual. From the time you get up in the morning until the time you retire at night, you do hundreds of things the same way every day – the way you shower, dress, eat breakfast, check your phone, brush your teeth, drive or commute to work, organise your desk, shop at the supermarket, or clean your bedroom or your house.

One of my mantras that I use most often on my podcast is: 'Tell me what you do every day, and I'll tell you where you'll be in a year'. The reason I use it so often is that it is applicable to everything we do. Tell or show me how you eat every day and the food choices you make, and I'll tell you how your body composition will look in a year.

For example, if you are consistently eating highly processed sugary food devoid of nutrients, there's a pretty good chance that you're going to be carrying around a spare tyre by this time next year. Remember the example of Martha from the chapter on 'The Compound Effect' earlier in the book.

The same goes for your personal or romantic relationships. If you walk through the door every single day and take out the day's frustration on your loved ones, how strong do you think those relationships will be in a year, not to mention five or ten years? You don't decide your future; you decide your habits, and your habits decide your future.

The beauty of habits is that once you recognise you've created an unsupportive or 'bad' habit, you can change it. It's not necessarily that easy to change, and the deeper engrained it is or the longer you've been doing it, the more difficult it is to change, but it can be done.

I categorise habits into supportive (good) and unsupportive (bad). I see supportive habits as those that get me closer to my end goal every single day. They feed into my four quadrants. If a current habit isn't moving me closer to a 9/10 in a specific quadrant, then I look at ways to break or change it.

For example, when I first wanted to get my body fat low enough to see my abs, I had the habit of going out and drinking alcohol three nights a week, and it wasn't helping my end goal. Therefore, I changed my actions to map onto that new ambition.

The first thing I did was write my goal down and put it somewhere I could see every single day. In my case, it was on my bedroom locker so I could see it every night before I went to bed and every morning when I woke up.

I also wrote it in the first person – 'I have 10% body fat and can see my abs clearly'. That way, I was conditioning my mind to believe that I was already in possession of that particular thing and was just waiting for reality to catch up to that end vision.

I know once I take the correct action steps, hitting the goal becomes inevitable. The time scale may change (adjust the timeline, not the goal) or the actual end goal may change or evolve (always give yourself permission to change your mind), but 99 out of 100 times, this is my process. I'm aware how 'woo-woo' and New Age that sounds, but I've done it like that for years. It has become a belief system I hold because of all the benefits that have manifested as a result. Feel free to do it your way, but here are some examples of my previous goals I listed on my bedroom locker:

1. I have 10% body fat and can see my abs clearly

In 2009, I set that goal at the age of twenty-one while I was at university. I hit my target after five weeks.

2. I step on stage for a bodybuilding show and am at my absolute best

I did this in 2014 and finished fourth at my first-ever show.

3. I have a thriving online fitness business that serves thousands of people a year

I set the goal in 2015 when I was moving my 1:1 personal training business online.

4. *The Fitness Mindset* is a #1 bestseller

My first book, *The Fitness Mindset*, hit the Amazon bestseller list within twenty-four hours of its release and stayed there for sixteen consecutive weeks. I set this goal in 2017.

5. I ran six back-to-back marathons in the Sahara

I achieved that goal in April 2018.

For giving up alcohol to get my body fat low enough to achieve my goal, I tried to find ways to change the habit. At the time, I figured I had two options. One: go cold turkey and just give up alcohol for four to six weeks and see if it helps. Two: gradually reduce my intake week by week – go from drinking three nights a week to two, and so on, in order to see how my body responded. If my body fat got low enough with two nights a week of drinking, I would have found my minimum effective dose (MED) – how much I can drink to get my body fat to a specific level.

Self-awareness is the key in choosing the strategy, as some people do better with option one and others do better with option two. I've always been an 'all or nothing' person and don't do great with moderation, so I committed to abstain from alcohol for six full weeks. At the time, by supplementing the strategy with good nutrition and training, my body fat actually went to single digits in just under five weeks. I had hit my target.

When trying to achieve any goal, it's worth asking the question: 'Should I go cold turkey or pursue moderation?' The answer is subjective. If you have a Type A 'all or nothing' personality like me, then it's probably best to go cold turkey on most bad habits. If you're on the other end of the spectrum, then reducing your intake gradually is probably going to be a better strategy. I am often asked how I know if I should go cold turkey or do moderation; instead of explaining it in detail, I want to introduce you to two people, Mary and Carl.

Mary and Carl are a couple on a journey to lose some body fat. They have decent nutrition and training habits; both go to the gym a few times a week and eat mostly nutrient-dense food, vegetables, fruits and wholegrains. But they have the same problem – both *love* chocolate! They are aware that their love of chocolate is probably the main hindrance in losing the desired amount of body fat and want to create a new habit that supports their new end goal – lowering body fat.

Mary, as we know, has an incredible sweet tooth. It's worth adding that she is known to her friends as 'Mary Moderation' (okay, not really, but the nickname helps us to remember the point). Anyway, the thought of not having a small bit of chocolate every day makes her physically anxious. Having a chocolate bar at lunchtime is the food highlight of her day, and she looks forward to it every morning. The thought of giving it up or waiting a full week for it makes life unbearable for her (again, I'm being dramatic but stick with me here).

In this case, Mary is probably going to be better off eating a little bit of chocolate every day and factoring it into her nutritional strategy. If she manages her calorie and food intake, she can adjust it to fit in a daily bar. As long as she's not consuming too many calories (calorie surplus) and she's eating high-quality nutrient-dense food, despite a chocolate bar every day, her body fat will gradually come down. Such a strategy is going to allow her to adhere to her nutritional strategy over the long term, creating a habit that allows her to continually reduce her body fat until she's happy with how she looks.

On the other hand, Carl, known to his friends as 'Carl Cold Turkey' (just go with me, folks), is a bit more extreme by nature. He wants to get his body fat down as well but looks at Mary and thinks, 'How does she do that? I couldn't eat a small amount of chocolate every day. If I did, the floodgates would open, and I would want to eat the whole box! Besides, I'd rather not have any all week and then have as much as I want on Saturday.'

Mary feels the opposite. She looks at Carl and thinks, 'I couldn't go a whole week without chocolate. I don't know how he does it?' Sound familiar?

If you have ever tried to lose weight, drop body fat or even build muscle, you're familiar with such a scenario in some form. Again, it may be with another food or drink choice, but the idea is generally the same.

At this juncture, you will also connect more with Mary or Carl and think one way is better than the other. In the context of getting body fat down, the reality is that both strategies work. Yes, the tactics may differ, but both work. Mary has to keep her calories in check each day to factor in her chocolate bar. Carl, on the other hand, is more likely to reduce his calorie intake on his 'chocolate day' and possibly do a hard workout around it to burn the sugars he's consuming. Regardless, both strategies work. Understanding what tactics you should employ is down to your personality type.

I resonate more with Carl because that's my personality type. As my friend Anna always tells me, 'You don't have a sweet tooth, Brian. You have sweet teeth,' and that's exactly how I am. I would rather go six days without chocolate and then have two or three big bars watching a movie on a Saturday night. I struggle and have always struggled with moderation, so I use this self-awareness to double down on tactics that work better for me. You may be the complete opposite. It's not about copying me or anybody else but about finding what works best for you and then applying that. Afterwards, the beauty of the compound effect starts to kick in.

Dealing with negative people

It's easy to think that the strategies of moderation and cold turkey just apply to fitness or nutrition; but if you think so, you're wrong. You may apply the same strategies if you are trying to weed negative people out of your life. Some work better with a full-cut approach – you identify the negative people who are consciously or subconsciously hindering your progress to become a better person or are always knocking you down, and in one fell swoop, you disconnect from them. No more hanging around with them, no more giving weighted attention to their opinions and no more attaching meaning to the words they throw at you. I did this years ago, and it was the best decision I ever made.

True, you cannot physically remove yourself from some people. It's significantly harder to cut out a father, a mother, brother, a sister or even a work colleague or a boss you see every day, but, in a lot of cases, you can control how much weight you give to their words. Even now, I interact with some of my biggest detractors, the people who knocked me down and told me I'd never amount to anything. They still question what I do and why I do it and project their own insecurities and inadequacies onto me, but I picture those words like water hitting my head. Yes, you feel it initially; then it just flows down the side of your face – no weight, no wounds.

This is also a point I can receive significant pushback on, and I will address this now. The above suggestion may resonate with some of you, and those lines will be your catalyst for change. Others may resist it and tell themselves the story: 'But it's my mum or my dad or my brother or my sister'. It may even be followed by 'Yes, they're horrible to me or never believed in me, but what can I do?'

You may still be able to spend time with those detractors and negative people, but the danger is probably in the dose. If you spend 80% of your day around such people, it's unlikely you're going to be happy or productive. You may be able to handle such people 5% of the time, 10% of the time or even 20% of the time. Similar to the chocolate bar, it's not the chocolate bar in isolation that's stopping you from losing body fat. As I mentioned, a small bar every day may even help you with your fat-loss goals; but if you eat ten chocolate bars every day, your body fat is probably going to increase and not decrease. The time you spend with negative and unsupportive people is the same. Audit your network and ensure your inner circle is a good one. After that, it's about making sure that your habits are created by design and not by default.

Habits by design, not by default

The great news is that building supportive habits frees up your mind while your body goes on automatic. For example, I drive two hours every day to the gym by choice. My business is online, so I can work from my home where I actually have a fully equipped gym. But the intentionally planned drive allows me to do two hours of audio-learning every day in the form of a podcast or audiobooks.

I do the same thing when I'm preparing meals or walking the dog. I call this 'hacking dead time' – using time that's normally spent doing something mindless (listening to music, daydreaming, etc) to consume something that supports you in the quadrant you are most focused on right now. In my mid-twenties, when I was travelling the world as a professional fitness model and bodybuilder, most of my audio-learning was based on training and nutrition. As my priorities shifted to business, I started to consume more audiobooks on that subject.

A question I ask myself is, 'Is this particular habit or thing I'm doing repeatedly moving me closer or further away from my end goal?' It is a simple question, but I still use it to this day when making decisions. I found that listening to music on my morning commute took me further from my end goal and I wasn't improving. Listening to audiobooks and informative podcasts, on the other hand, educated me on my 'unknown unknowns' and started to fill the gaps in my knowledge, which compounded over several years.

You can effectively turn your car into a library on wheels, and once the compound effect kicks in, you will start to see things changing for the better. I purchased a brand-new car in 2016 and haven't turned on the radio since I bought it. I don't even know how to work it. The radio is automatically linked to my phone, and as soon as I start the car in the morning, the podcast or audiobook that I have been listening to continues playing on Bluetooth.

To be clear, I'm not asking you to quit listening to music or watching entertainment programmes. On the contrary, it's important to have some downtime or 'mindless' time factored into your day, and I discuss this in detail in the 'Rewire Your Mental Health' chapter. I mostly rely on live sports or movies for my downtime, but music or a TV show serves the same purpose. I generally apply the 80:20 Pareto principle here.

The Pareto principle, named after the Italian civil engineer, economist and sociologist Vilfredo Pareto, was originally applied to describing the distribution of wealth in a society, in line with the trend that a large portion of wealth is held by a small fraction of the population. This rule states that, for example, 80% of the wealth of a particular society is held by 20% of its population. However, this formula can work equally well in planning how you spend your day.

I use 80% of my 'dead' time for driving, commuting, prepping food, utility shopping and consuming something that helps support my life in a meaningful way. The other 20% of my time is for entertainment – watching live sports or TV shows, listening to music, etc. If you commute or drive for one to two hours every day and devote 80% of that time to listening to music, don't be surprised that nothing in your life is changing for the better. Remember the example of Linda from 'The Compound Effect' chapter earlier in the book.

Just try it for a month. Whatever be your priority right now – strengthening your mindset, looking after your fitness or health, building your business – while on your morning and evening commute, listen to or read (if you take public transport) something that educates you on that area of your life. I started doing this in 2013, and it's one of the best decisions I ever made. Once it becomes a habit, it feels weird not doing it!

Habits are so powerful and determine so much of how our lives turn out, but the bad news is that we can also become locked into habits that don't serve us – unconscious self-defeating behaviour patterns that inhibit our growth and limit our success. What's worse is that such unsupportive or 'bad' habits can become so subconscious that we don't even realise we have them.

Creating a bad habit

The first audiobook I ever listened to was *The Power of Habit* by Charles Duhigg, and the book changed the way I looked at everything I did in my life.[1]

At the time, I was working as a primary school teacher in West London and had picked up quite a few bad habits. One was coming home after work every day, plopping down in the same chair and numbing out to the TV while devouring two or three chocolate bars. Two months into the routine, my jeans were getting a little too tight for comfort and I was losing my shape. I had created a bad habit.

---

[1] C Duhigg (2012) *The Power of Habit*. New York: Random House.

Creating positive habits and breaking negative ones

In *The Fitness Mindset*, I spoke about the 'cue–routine–reward' system of habits. To change a habit, you need to change one of the components of the 'cue–routine–reward' system. The cue is the actual situation or 'trigger' for an action. For me, the trigger was coming home every day after work. The routine is what one does after the cue. In my case, the routine was taking out two or three bars of chocolate from the cupboard, plopping down in my chair and watching the same shows. The reward is the endorphin release or the 'happy feeling' one experiences when eating sugar or chocolate.

As soon as I realised the habit was affecting me negatively, I put plans in place to change one of the components. For me, the trigger or cue of coming home from work was always going to be the same; therefore, I changed the routine. Instead of reaching for chocolate bars in the cupboard, I left a pre-packed gym bag beside the front door. I would come home (cue or trigger), pick up my gym bag (new routine), and the reward came via the endorphin release from exercise.

Your habits determine your outcomes. Successful people don't just drift to the top. Getting to the top requires focused action, personal discipline and considerable energy every day to make things happen. The habits you develop from this day forward will ultimately determine how your future unfolds. Your words to yourself are powerful, and one of the self-talk mindset rewirings I've successfully implemented over the years has two components to it.

The first one is being completely honest about my bad habits. It took me a while to realise that lying to myself about my bad habits just makes them compound worse over time. As I said earlier, if you don't deal with a problem when it's small enough to be solved, you deserve to deal with the mess when it grows.

The truth is you can only bang your head against a wall so many times before you start wondering why it hurts. Hence, rule #1 – don't fool yourself. If you have a bad habit, own it.

The second component is adding the words 'up until now' to the end of every sentence about an unsupportive habit. When I first decided to run through the Sahara, the negative story that replayed in my mind was, 'You're not good enough, or you're not brave enough'. This way of thinking had become so common for me over the years that it had become hardwired. I had a bad habit of speaking down to myself. It wasn't until I replaced the words 'I'm not good enough' or 'I'm not brave enough' with 'I haven't been good enough' or 'I haven't been brave enough… up until now' that my mind started to open to new ways of seeing how I could achieve my end goal. Instead of my mind shutting down by taking the path of least resistance, something that happens automatically when we tell ourselves we can't do something, the images of who I had to become in order to hit my target flashed in my mind.

My new internal dialogue was something like this: 'Okay, cool, you haven't been good enough or fit enough to run six back-to-back marathons until now.

Great. What do you have to do now to become good enough?' Suddenly, the answers started to pop into my head: 'I need to run more; I need to condition my body and mind so that I can withstand the pain. I need to reframe the pain as a positive thing and know that each step gets me closer to my goal.'

The next step was dealing with the fear: 'Okay, what's that nagging fear, Brian? You don't think you're brave enough. How can you become brave enough?' Again, the answers started to pop into my mind from nowhere: 'Remember all those other times you were afraid and you did it anyway. Remember you were scared to do public speaking once and now you do it for a living. Think about your daughter and how scared you were before she was born, but that turned out to be the best thing that ever happened to you.'

I had to hijack my negative self-talk and replace it with something better. Five months later, I ran six back-to-back marathons through the Sahara in Morocco. The fear never goes away. You feel it and do it anyway, but the self-talk also never goes away (for me, at least). It just gets quieter and quieter or you learn to hijack it quicker. The more goals I set and achieve, the quieter that voice tends to get.

If you can get to the root of your self-talk and hijack it so that it doesn't paralyse you, you can achieve anything!

Take actions to develop better habits

One of the problems encountered by people with poor habits is that the results of their bad habits usually don't show up until much later in life. My bad habit of talking down to myself manifested itself in my failure to makes changes, as I didn't believe I was good enough to make them. It was a failure of omission, really – the results of the actions I didn't take. The more I avoided the things I was afraid of, the more hardwired the habit became. As I said in the 'Rewire Fear' chapter, the same works in reverse now. I consciously attack the things I'm afraid of because that's the habit I want to instil in myself and become automatic.

When you develop a chronic bad habit, life will eventually give you the consequences. I was twenty-four before I started to question these self-limiting beliefs and spent the next six or seven years trying to iron them out and rewire them. When I realised that regardless of whether I liked the consequences of my habits, life delivered them to me all the same, I felt the need to find a way to break the cycle.

The fact is when you keep on doing things a certain way, you will continue to get predictable results. If you always skip working out and continue to make poor food choices, your health and waistline will pay the price for that. If you repeatedly ignore the people closest to you and don't give them the attention or love they need, then don't be surprised when they turn around and leave you in five, ten or even twenty years.

Negative habits breed negative consequences. Positive habits breed positive results.

There are just two action steps for changing your habits. The first step is to make a list of all the bad habits that keep you unproductive or may negatively impact your future. I find it helpful to ask my inner circle about my 'blind spots' as well – the habits I've created that I haven't necessarily noticed or I'm wilfully blind to.

Note that being informed about your blind spots by another person can be difficult, but remember it's better to be punched hard by the truth than kissed softly by a lie. I also tend to share my end goals with the people closest to me as they can keep me accountable if I'm misallocating my time, energy or resources towards something else that isn't my top priority at the moment.

For example, when I was writing my first book *The Fitness Mindset*, I would tell my inner circle the dates by which I wanted each section completed. If I tried to replace my 'writing time' (normally the first two to three hours of the day) with something else, they would call me out on it and help me shift my focus back towards my main goal.

The second step is to make a list of your most common unsupportive habits. Here are some of mine from an old journal that I kept:

1. Procrastinating

If left to my default mode, I'm probably the world's worst procrastinator. I generally find that the 'eat the frog' principle works well here. Mark Twain said that if you eat a frog first thing in the morning, the rest of the day can only get better. In other words, if you do the least interesting or the most daunting or challenging of tasks in the morning, the rest of the day will be better.

I normally do my most 'anxiety-driven' or 'non-negotiable creative' tasks first thing in the morning. This is normally when I'm at my freshest and my will power is at its highest. Anxiety-driven tasks are generally the things I really don't want to do – writing or replying to emails, creating PDFs, among others. My non-negotiable creative tasks are things that move my fulfilment quadrant forward – writing a book, creating podcasts, among others.

2. Spending money before having it

If you've ever bought something on credit or used up money allocated for other purposes because 'it's payday next week', then you know what I'm talking about here.

This was my worst financial habit for years. I would buy things I didn't really need all the while thinking 'Sure, I'm getting paid next week' and then overspend every month. I always wondered why I had no savings come the end of the year. I broke this bad habit by adopting the 'pay yourself first' approach. This meant that a portion of my income – a fixed percentage – automatically went into my savings each month. I never see it; I don't get to spend it.

When my income goes up, my savings go up with it proportionately. I never deviate from the percentage either. The alternative for me was that my lifestyle would match my pay increase. When I was an employee, if my wages went up, I bought a nicer car or a new TV. Now, although I'm no longer an employee and run my own company, I still save the same percentage of my income every month. Now, it's just habit.

3. Getting up too late in the morning

My proclivity to sleep is a habit that never served me. When I started to win the battle of the mind over mattress, everything else throughout the day felt significantly easier.

4. Working too late into the evening

I used to work right until bedtime. The habit not only negatively affected my sleep but also wreaked havoc in my personal relationships. I could never 'switch off'. For example, while playing with my daughter, I would be thinking about the work task I had to finish, and when I was working on that task, I would feel guilty I wasn't spending enough time with my daughter.

I broke this habit using two different strategies: One, focusing on the WIN or repeating the mantra 'Be here now' for several seconds until my mind refocused. Once I did that, I could go back to making a jigsaw puzzle with my daughter or writing a section for the blog article while being fully present in the moment.

Two, having a non-negotiable switch-off period each night. Except on the days I'm interviewing or working with people in different time zones across the globe, I generally finish work every day at 6pm. After that, no emails, no social media, no messages, nothing, it all gets shut down at 6pm.

Wrapping up work at my non-negotiable switch-off period helped me to not only sleep better but also improve my work quality. Parkinson's Law describes this anomaly better: 'Work expands to fill the time available for its completion'. If you only have two hours or four hours to finish the same task, in most cases, I bet it will take you the full time to complete.

Don't be like me and choose to be a 'busy fool' and confuse movement with progress. Being busy and being productive are completely different things. Being busy means you have a lot of work to do; being productive means you're getting a lot of work done. Finish your work each day and then switch off. You'll be a better parent, partner or just a less-stressed individual because of it. I apply this exact principle to my workouts and training. In most cases, a twenty-minute high-intensity workout is better than a three-hour session where you're taking ten-minute breaks between exercises. Always focus on the quality, not the quantity.

5. Choosing work over children

I had always prided myself on being a good dad. Yet, when my daughter was about eighteen months old, I realised my actions weren't mapping onto that ambition. I would tell people and, worse, tell myself that my daughter and family were always more important to me than work, but my actions didn't map onto that.

If I was working on a deadline, I always prioritised my work. It wasn't until I had a dream one night that it all changed. In the dream, I saw an older me sitting behind my desk at home, typing away on my laptop. Then, my daughter comes running into the room, jumping up and down with a picture she had drawn, screaming, 'Daddy, Daddy, Daddy, look'. But I just ignored her, staring straight at my screen. I remember seeing a tear roll down her face and the picture dropping. It was a crayon drawing of me and her at the playground I take her to every weekend. My dream self was looking at this picture and shouting, 'Pay attention to her, you idiot! You're never going to get this moment again!'

I woke up seconds later dripping in sweat. The dream was so vivid that I still remember it years later. It sounds weird even reading back now, but at the time, it made me realise that my actions weren't mapping onto my ambition.

My 97-year-old rule, discussed in the last chapter of the book, came to me a few months later. On reflection, I feel that the image I saw in the dream sowed the seed for that principle. Now I don't have to dream it anymore. I can just turn to the 97-year-old rule and ask, 'What would my 97-year-old self on my deathbed regret more? Not sending that email and going to a last-minute business meeting or missing my daughter's first

Christmas recital?' It's simple when you put it like that, but your actions speak louder than your words. If your actions aren't mapping onto your ambition, then you need to change your actions or change your ambition. 2+2 never equals 5 no matter how many times you add it up. I fooled myself into thinking it could, and I'm thankful to my subconscious mind and the dream for metaphorically finally waking me up.

A few years later, I received direct feedback that I was on the right path. The day I came back from the Sahara, I had been gone for ten days and had over 900 emails in my inbox. I also had clients who needed to be replied to and appearances to make. The day after I got back, I remember waking up at 9am, and as I was packing my bags to go to the city for work, Holly, who was nearly three at the time, saw me. She came over and asked, 'Can you please stay with me today?' It felt like the dream had come back to me for the first time in a year. I took out my phone, cancelled all my meetings and told my operations manager to reply to emails and apologise to clients, but it would be another day before I would be back to them. We spent the entire day playing with princess dolls, watching Disney movies and gorging on ice cream. I've never made a better decision in my entire life.

Never forget that you will always prioritise what you value, but sometimes you just need a little reminder of what the real valuables in your life are. Money, emails, work projects are all important in their own respect, but when you're ninety-seven and on your death bed, you're never going to regret not working more. You're never going to regret not sending emails. You will regret not looking up at the picture and hugging your child. You will regret cancelling the dinner with your mum or dad because of a work meeting. Remember, not everything that can be counted counts and not everything that counts can be counted.

When it comes to bad habits, your list may be completely different from mine; you may have bad habits of talking over people, answering the phone in the middle of dinner conversations or having fast-food meals twice a week. The key is identifying the bad habits, then owning them. Yes, it's how you've lived with your bad habits until now, but now it's time to change it. Once you have identified your negative habits, the second step is to choose better, more productive success habits and develop systems that will help support them.

For example, if you eat healthily you've likely built healthy habits around food – what you put in your shopping basket or what you order in restaurants. The same thing happens if you eat unhealthily; you make different choices automatically.

Even though we develop most of our habits unconsciously, by modelling our parents, responding to environmental or cultural associations, or developing coping mechanisms, we can consciously decide to change them. Reflect on how deeply your habits are rooted and then put the plan together to create new positive ones in their place.

Becoming self-aware of your negative behaviours,

patterns and habits isn't always easy; that's why reading certain books is crucial as they can 'point' things out we may have missed or failed to see.

As I mentioned in the opening chapter, I try and live my life by internalising that there are only three ways to look at most of the things in my life: 1) the things I know; 2) the things I don't know; and 3) the things I don't know that I don't know. I used and still use books, podcasts and the instructions of the right people on social media to bridge the gap between all three.

The story of the boy and the tree

The Power of Habit by Charles Duhigg brought me to the understanding that I was living in a pattern without even realising it. The book brought this to my attention and put me in a much more positive place mentally and physically. However, reading the story about the pupil and the wise teacher made me realise that some habits are harder to change than others.

The story of the boy and the tree comes from my first book, *The Fitness Mindset*, and goes like this. Taking a stroll through a forest with a young boy, a teacher stops before a tiny tree. 'Pull up that sapling', the teacher instructs the boy, pointing at a newly emerging sprout from the earth. The boy pulls it up easily with his fingers. 'Now pull up that one', orders the teacher, indicating a more well-rooted sapling that has grown to about knee length. With a little effort, the boy yanks the plant, and it springs free, uprooted. 'And now, this one', says the teacher, nodding towards a more developed evergreen as tall as the young boy. With great effort, throwing all his weight and strength into the task, using sticks and stones, the boy unearths the stubborn roots, getting the tree loose. 'Now', the teacher says, 'I'd like you to pull this one up'. The young boy follows the teacher's gaze and sees a mighty oak so tall he can scarcely see the top. Knowing the struggle he had just gone through pulling up a much smaller tree, he simply tells the teacher, 'I am sorry, but I can't'. The teacher exclaims, 'My son, you have just demonstrated the power habits will have over your life! The older they are, the bigger they get; the deeper the roots grow, the harder they are to uproot. Some get big, with roots so deep, you may hesitate to try to uproot them.'

Small bad habits like the one I mentioned earlier are easy to change by understanding the 'cue–routine–reward' system. By just changing one of the components of the system, you can effectively change your habits. Some habits are harder to break than others; some have 'deeper roots'. For example, if you have never felt confident about the way you look or have been overweight your entire life, you're not going to change one thing and wake up lean or full of confidence overnight.

Deep-rooted habits are more difficult to change, but the small things you do every day will allow you to change these particular habits. I have worked with people who have been overweight their entire lives, some for more than twenty years. They get frustrated when they're not lean after two weeks of following a diet and workout programme. If I told you I wanted to learn Spanish but wanted to be fluent in two weeks, what would you tell me? It's probably not possible, right? But what if I said I wanted to be fluent in six, twelve or eighteen months? Then, my desire becomes a lot more realistic. Breaking bad habits is the same; you're not going to break a habit you've had for five, ten or twenty years in two weeks. But, by taking the right steps, you can break it at six or twelve months and then forever. After that, it's rewiring how you see failure and understanding that failure is not an end product but feedback.

10

Rewire Failure as Feedback

What failure can tell us

> 'A good person dyes events with his own col-
> our... and turns whatever happens to his own
> benefit.'
> — Seneca

Imagine the sound of a footstep. If I asked you, 'What
does a footstep mean?' you would probably answer,
'It doesn't mean anything to me'. Well, let's think about
that. If you're walking along a busy street, you hear so
many footsteps that you don't even hear them distinctly.
In that situation, they don't have any effective meaning.
But what if you're home alone late at night, and you
hear footsteps downstairs? A moment later, you hear
the steps moving towards you. Do the footsteps have
meaning then? They sure do. The same signal (the
sound of footsteps) will have many different meanings
depending on what it has meant to you in similar
situations in the past.

Your experience may provide you with a context for the signal and thus determine whether it relaxes or frightens you. For example, if you've just started a new workout programme and feel a little sore the next day, you will feel pretty good that you pushed your body to its limit, and you know that the pain you are currently feeling is ultimately moving you towards a particular end goal – such as getting fitter, losing weight or building muscle. But, if you felt that same pain and immediately thought that you might have a cancerous tumour, you would certainly feel differently about the situation. You felt pain in both cases, but the meanings you attached to that pain were completely different. Thus, the meaning of any experience in life depends upon the frame in which we place it. If you change the frame, the meaning changes instantly. Over the years, I've learned that one of the most effective tools for personal change is learning how to put the best frames on any experience.

It took me a long time to cultivate the skills to get out of my own way when looking to hit the targets I set for myself. But the one thing that has supported me more than anything else is the rewiring of my mindset towards failure in any given situation.

When you realise that 'failure' is essentially feedback and just one more way that didn't work, you see that it has given you crucial information on how to tweak the formula going forward. Every failure gets you one step closer to the end goal.

Suppose you've had three terrible relationships

that ended with your partner cheating on you. Good. Now you have feedback that something is wrong in your selection process or you're mindlessly going after people who aren't right for you. Great. Own that. View the failure up to this point as feedback and change the decisions you're making in that area of your life. In this example, first you may have to make a list of all the positive qualities you want in a partner. Next, ask yourself how you can deserve that kind of person. Once you stop reliving the same mistakes over and over again, you can change the outcome.

I spoke earlier about going through the back of my couch to find money for a bus ride after my third attempt at starting my business had failed. That experience has allowed me to work with many entrepreneurs to help them avoid the same mistakes. That's a textbook example of the role our perceptions play in our success or failure overcoming the things that oppose us. It's one thing not to be overwhelmed, discouraged or upset by obstacles, but it's another thing to genuinely see that most great opportunities grow from the seeds of failures.

Barcelona ultramarathon

When I was training to run 230 km through the Arctic Circle, I signed up for a 76km ultramarathon in Barcelona several months beforehand. It was technically my first-ever one-day ultramarathon, and I was worried about the distance to be covered. Although

I had run six back-to-back marathons through the Sahara, I didn't feel particularly strong going into the event. The day before the race, I found out that the area to be covered was 90% forest and the start of the run included a run to the top of Mount Tibidabo, the tallest mountain in the Serra de Collserola.

I wasn't too worried about the forest terrain or even the incline run up the mountain, but I was concerned about the navigation. My mum used to joke when I was a kid that I'd get lost on the way from my bedroom to the kitchen if I didn't have such a keen sense of smell, but I'm genuinely very poor with directions and navigation. This is partly due to a lack of interest in upskilling in this area and partly because I've never felt the need to improve owing to the invention of Google Maps and satellite navigation. Still, on this particular excursion, my Google Maps didn't work, and I did in fact in get lost.

Around 40 km into the 76km race, I took a wrong turn and ended up at a different checkpoint. Ultramarathons normally have checkpoints one has to go through at each race. Generally, food and water are available at the checkpoints, and they track you electronically at each one to make sure you don't get lost. The woman at this checkpoint told me I had taken the wrong way and I needed to double back 10 km to go through the correct checkpoint. It had been raining in Barcelona for the previous two weeks, and I was soaked from head to toe. I was tired, frustrated and angry that I had taken the wrong route. I also knew if I didn't make the

10 km in less than 50 minutes, I would be timed out of the entire race. So I quit. I ran back to the start line, which was about 12 km from the incorrect checkpoint, and happily got my backpack and headed to my hotel.

I arrived back at the hotel room and was happy that the race was over. I showered, ate and relaxed on the bed. Then, the remorse of having quit the race hit me. True, I might not have made the cut-off and would have timed out anyway, but I made the conscious decision to quit the race.

I had flown down to Barcelona with a pair of shorts and road shoes, thinking I was going to run 76 km through the city. I hadn't been prepared, and I also hadn't even fully committed to finishing the race. When I was only 25 km into the race, I had already been having such a miserable time (my road shoes wouldn't get any grip in the terrain, and I had to walk large sections of the mountain) that I would have quit then and there if given an excuse.

The whole experience ate at me for about three weeks. I was disappointed in myself for quitting. I was annoyed at the race directors for mixing up the checkpoints (my own projected annoyance), but truthfully, I was angry at myself for not being prepared and committed to finishing beforehand.

When I flew to the Sahara six months earlier, I had been committed to finishing or leaving the desert in a helicopter ambulance if I had to. As preparation for the marathon, I had consistently run 50–100 km every week and had been as physically prepared as I could have been prior to the event. I had done none of that for the Barcelona ultramarathon. On race day, I had just arrived in the city, thinking I'd breeze through it. I told myself, 'Man, you ran six to back-to-back marathons through the Sahara. You can easily run 76 km in your sleep'. As the saying goes, pride always comes before the fall.

As if the universe was trying to send me a message, the book I had picked to read that week was Robert Greene's *The 33 Strategies for War*.[1] I've always been a history geek, but a chapter of the book was titled 'Lose Battles, But Win the War'.

Suddenly, I reframed the failure in Barcelona as a battle, which it was. I had scheduled it as a preparation run for the Arctic Circle marathon. I paired that thinking with the uncomfortable realisation that I couldn't go to the Arctic (or anywhere again) with the attitude I had in Barcelona. Past successes mean nothing if your current attitude is wrong. The experience taught me to never go unprepared for anything again and to either commit fully to the goal or not do it at all. In February 2019, I ran 230 km through the Arctic Circle. My success at the Arctic grew from the seed of failure in Barcelona. The failure had taught me lessons as valuable as my success in the desert. Failure is not an end product; it's feedback.

I'm aware that seeing failure as feedback is something we are not hardwired to do. But after you have

---

1   R Greene (2006) *The 33 Strategies for War*. New York: Penguin Group.

controlled your emotions or surrendered the attachment to 'how it should have been' or 'what others will think', you can see objectively what is right in front of your eyes – the obstacle is really an opportunity.

As American writer Laura Ingalls Wilder put it, 'There is good in everything, if only we look for it'.[2] Yet, we can be so bad at looking. We close our eyes to the gift in front of us – direct feedback on how to get closer to our end goal.

If you hate your job, you have direct feedback on what line of work you probably shouldn't be in. If you're in a co-dependent and soul-destroying relationship, then you have feedback on what to avoid the next time. If you're not happy with the way you look, you have direct feedback that you probably need a new nutritional, training or lifestyle strategy. In this case, it may also be feedback that you're focusing on the wrong things and letting negativity bias take control.

To digress for a minute, as someone who has worked in the fitness industry for years, I've seen some of the most objectively attractive women and men walk around with their shoulders slouched and their heads down because they could only focus on the 5% of them that wasn't 'perfect' – chubby legs, a little back fat or small arms.

Remember, what you focus on is what will expand, and if you focus on the 5% of what you're unhappy with, then that will become the 95% of your attention.

---

2   R Holiday (2006) *The Daily Stoic*. London: Profile Books.

Again, this is rewiring your mindset. If you're not happy with something that can be changed, then change it. As I mentioned earlier, if you're unhappy where you are, then move. You are not a tree! If the thing that you're focusing on cannot be changed, then you're wasting energy on something out of your control.

Why don't you cry when it rains outside?

There's a reason we don't sit and dwell on the weather when it's raining outside. Yes, we may complain we're going to get wet on our commute or maybe have to cancel or change plans, but we don't sit and mope around all day that it's raining. We cannot change it, and we know this. Yet, we don't apply the same thinking to things like raising our kids, going for a new job or getting into a better relationship. All we can do is set up our lives to allow good things to happen and not worry about the rest.

Suppose you're worried your kids won't turn out okay. Then focus on being present with them, teach them as much as you can about how the world works and then trust you did a good enough job. If you're worried about going for a new occupation, then learn the skills and develop the relationships or networks that make you hireable. If you're afraid to get into a better relationship because you feel you don't deserve it, then start looking into all the ways of developing your self-worth. But for your own sake, don't dwell on the things out of your control. That's like complaining about why you can't stop the rain. Yes, there's always a possibility that it may rain, but it's a hell of a lot easier to carry an umbrella than to sit at home and wish for it to stop. Control the things that are in your control, create environments that allow good things to happen and then stop worrying about the rest.

In most cases, it's not what actually happens to us that's the problem anyway. Our preconceptions are the problem. We think that things should or need to be a certain way, so when they're not, we naturally assume we are at a disadvantage or we'd be wasting our time to pursue an alternative course. In reality, it's all fair game, and every situation is an opportunity for us to act.

Even while writing this book, I lost a full chapter twice when creating my first draft. One was the chapter on self-sabotage, so I re-wrote the whole thing. I had to keep telling myself that it was meant to be deleted from my laptop and now I had an opportunity to make it twice as good as before. The irony of losing a chapter on self-sabotage is not lost on me either. Sometimes, it doesn't even matter if you believe it at the time, but if you repeat something to yourself enough times and focus your energy and attention on it, it will expand and become a reality.

Of course, you will want to avoid something negative if you can, but life doesn't always work out that way, and rewiring your mindset is a valuable tool in your toolkit. Sports psychologists conducted a study on elite athletes who were stuck with some adversity or serious injury. Initially, each reported feeling isolation, emotional disruption and doubts of their athletic ability. Yet afterwards, each reported gaining a desire to help others, additional perspective and realisation of their own strengths.[3] Psychologists call this phenomenon 'adversarial growth' and 'post-traumatic growth'. 'That which doesn't kill us makes me stronger' is not a cliché but a fact for some people.

I compete in ultra-endurance events for the same reason. On top of the physical pain, which makes me psychologically stronger, I have to go to a dark place mentally to get through some of those events; every time I do, though, it gives me a fresh perspective on the things that are important to me – my family and my inner circle as well as serving others and focusing on those who will cry when I die.

The struggle against obstacles propels you to a new level of functioning. The extent of the struggle determines the extent of the growth. You don't need to run through the Sahara or undertake the Ironman Triathlon. Your struggle may be to go for a walk, jog or run after work (even when you know you're going to be tired) or setting that morning alarm ten minutes earlier so that you're not running out the door first thing every day. The obstacle or perceived obstacle is always an advantage. The real problem is any perceptions that prevent you from seeing this. Remember

---

3   D Fletcher, 'Psychological Resilience and Adversarial Growth in
     Sport and Performance', https://oxfordre.com/psychology/view/10
     .1093/acrefore/9780190236557.001.0001/acrefore-9780190236557-e-158

that we interject perspective into everything. Here are some of the personal issues of mine I've reframed and am now thankful for.

- When people are rude or disrespectful, I tell myself they're having a bad day or projecting their issues onto me. They also may not have the self-awareness to realise what they're doing. Why should I be mad about something when the other person isn't even aware they're doing it?
- When people put me down or tell me that I can't do something, I use it as the fuel for my fire. On the mornings I don't want to get up at 5am, I remember those words. Instead of lashing out at your detractors, let your actions speak louder than your words.
- When people are critical or question my ability or intelligence, I think to myself, 'Great, that lowers expectations. Low expectations are always easy to exceed.'

The above-mentioned are just some of my rewires. Think about the beliefs or thoughts that aren't supporting you and then flip them around. Nothing is good or bad; it's your attachment to it that determines how it makes you feel.

Face what isn't working

> 'Facts do not cease to exist because they are
> ignored.'
> — Aldous Huxley

It's important to bear in mind that failure is direct feedback on what isn't working, but that doesn't always translate to persevering in every hard situation. The reason having your ladder up against the right wall is so important is that every minor failure on a particular day gets you one more rung up the ladder. True, it might seem like you are going backwards at the time, like I was in Barcelona, but it's the figurative one step backwards for two steps forward.

If you know you're in the right relationship with the person you want to spend the rest of your life with, any fight or argument that needs to be had is a chance to make that relationship stronger. However, if you're in the wrong relationship and you know your ladder is against the wrong wall, then any fight or argument is feedback indicating that it may be time to change something.

The case of your job is exactly the same. If your ladder is against the right wall, even though the work deadlines are stressing you out right now, you know that when the work is complete you're going to be one step higher than when you started. That stress can make you stronger, but there will come a time when you have to face what isn't working.

If you are going to become the best version of

yourself, you have to get out of denial and face what isn't working in your life. This has also been one of my biggest struggles. It's so easy to disguise fear as practicality and concoct a story that justifies why you don't take that jump into the unknown, be it a job, a new relationship, or even improving your physical or mental health.

In this book, I've made several references to the importance of asking yourself questions, so here's another one: Is there some part of your life where you're playing 'ostrich with head in the sand'? Are you ignoring the physical world and what's going on around you because you don't want to face the truth? Do you defend or ignore how toxic your work environment is? Do you make excuses for your bad relationship? Are you in denial about your lack of energy, your excess weight, your ill health or your lack of physical fitness? Are you failing to acknowledge that your life has been on a downward spiral for the last six months? Are you putting off confronting an employee or employer who is not delivering or recognising your efforts?

The most successful people I've met over the past several years seem to have this one particular characteristic in common: they face their circumstances and reality head on. Yes, they heed the warning signs and take appropriate action, but they lean into the discomfort no matter how challenging a situation may be. Until recently, I spent too much of life ignoring reality and had to learn to rewire my thinking and model the people I looked up to most.

I've probably used every excuse one can think of when trying to get out of an uncomfortable situation – I'm too tired; it's too early; I'm sore; it's too hard; I can't commit to that right now; my dog needs a pedicure; the earth is orbiting the sun in a weird way. All excuses, but I learned a very valuable lesson doing ultra-endurance events. You can find an excuse, or you can find a way, but you can't do both. In Barcelona, I found excuses – it's too wet; it's not important; I don't have the right shoes. In the Sahara and the Arctic, it was the opposite. I separated real problems from perceived problems and just kept putting one foot in front of the other until I got to the respective finish lines. You can find an excuse, or you can find a way, but you can't do both.

Although the bad situations in our lives can be uncomfortable, embarrassing and painful, we often live with them, or, at worst, we wrap them in a story that justifies our actions. Most of the time, we don't even realise we are in denial. When I stopped fooling myself, I was able to make the necessary changes to improve my life. Here are some examples of what denial looked like for me:

- I can't do that – I'm not fit enough, fast enough or strong enough
- I can't talk to that person – I'm not smart enough, good-looking enough or witty enough
- It's none of my business or not my place to say – I shouldn't get involved
- I need this to help me relax – I numb my personal

issues with excessive alcohol, drugs, medication
or hours of watching mindless TV

Examples I frequently hear from other people are:

- It's just what guys/girls do
- They are just venting their frustration
- You know that's how they get when they're tired/
  drunk/stressed
- Everybody goes into credit card debt
- It's okay; everybody does it
- I'm sure they are going to pay me back
- I don't want to rock the boat
- I have to put in more hours at work if I want to
  get ahead
- I'll start an exercise programme or eating healthy
  when I have more time
- I just don't have time for that right now

Occasionally, we even make up reasons to convince
ourselves that something that is not working is working,
not realising that if we acknowledge the bad situation
sooner, it will be often less painful to resolve. Problems,
issues and dilemmas are like seeds. They're easy to
dig up when they've just been planted. If somebody
says something you dislike or belittles you in front of
your friends or work colleagues, it's a lot easier to pull
them aside right after or the next day (after you calm
down) and tell them how that comment made you feel.
If you don't, like a seed, it will grow and fester until it
becomes a lot harder to handle. The words or scenario

replay in your head, causing you unnecessary stress or insecurity, and you'll be in a constant state of worry any time that person walks into the room, fearing the same situation will occur again.

Confront the problem before it grows

When I lived in London and was working full time, I shared a house with three other men, all teachers. As we were young and single, our major interests were sports and partying. I was a little more into fitness than the others and always prioritised going to the gym before our Saturday nights out.

We always used to do 'pre-drinking' – having cheap drinks at our house before going to a bar or club – as we made very little money as teachers. During pre-drinks, we would always play games and have ten or twenty people over at our house.

On this one occasion, we were playing a general knowledge drinking game. Admittedly, at the time, my general knowledge was average but not great, as I didn't really start reading books until I was twenty-four or twenty-five years old. Although I possessed decent knowledge from teaching, my housemates, being older than me, were much more well informed. A question about geography came around, something to do with a European Union country name beginning with 'S' or 'T'. My housemate asked me the question, and I had no idea what the answer was. But it's what happened next that stuck with me for years.

When I told my housemate I didn't know the answer, he replied, 'You're a bit stupid for that one. I bet if it were a question about picking up a weight, you'd know' (in reference to having gone to the gym a few hours earlier). Everyone in the room chuckled, and then the turn went to the person beside me. At this point, if you've been reading the book in a linear order, you may recall that 'stupid' used to be one of my trigger words. That comment lit me up inside! I was furious, but I said nothing. For the next year and a half, I intentionally avoided spending any time with my housemate. I started staying over at my girlfriend's house a little more often and then eventually moved out completely. I never said a word about it.

I also never forgot what he had said. Six years later, he messaged me to come visit him when I was on a business trip in London. I actually dodged the meeting twice before I finally agreed to his third request. At this stage, I had left the teaching profession and was working with some of the world's leading fitness professionals. I had also just signed a deal for my first book and felt like a success. When I finally agreed to meet him, I embarrassingly remember thinking, 'I'll show you who's stupid now' as I went to his house wearing nice clothes and my fancy new watch.

I arrived at his front door, and we spoke for ten or twenty minutes before I brought up the comment he had made several years earlier. I broached it slowly, but then it came pouring out of me. He listened attentively and, unsurprisingly, he didn't even remember making the comment. At that moment, I realised I had let a great friendship go down the drain because I let an insecurity of mine project onto one of my closest friendships. He apologised profusely and admitted he never would have said it if he knew how badly it would affect me.

In *The Fitness Mindset*, I mentioned how we take the opinions of others and let them dictate the decisions we make, and we hold onto this anger or hate because we think it makes us feel better. There's an old saying that, 'Hating somebody is like drinking poison and expecting the other person to die'. Going back, if I had just brought my friend aside the following day and told him how small that comment made me feel, that seed would never have grown.

Pathetically, the reason I met up with my former housemate was to prove to him how wrong he had been. I let the seed of anger and hate build and build and build until that seed became a mighty oak tree. My friend didn't even remember what he had said, but I built it up in my own head.

It was a small problem that could have been solved with one conversation, but I let it escalate internally over the years. Although sometimes hate can be justified, in a lot of cases it's wasted energy. That was what I did in this particular situation, but feel free to learn from my mistakes. Also, if you care to know, I still keep in touch with that friend, and we remain close to this day. That entire situation was avoidable if I hadn't been such a cowardly victim and confronted it when it was small enough to be dealt with.

Deal with all your problems when they are small enough to be solved and don't let them grow.

Is your story holding you back?

A big part of getting out of denial is getting good at recognising bad situations and then deciding to do something about them. When I left my full-time teaching job, I had spent the previous two years telling myself that it wasn't practical to leave a full-time salary to become self-employed. My mind concocted stories about what could go wrong – 'What if I couldn't get any clients?' or 'What if I couldn't afford my rent or food?' My deep-rooted insecurities manifested in thoughts like, 'What would my friends or family think if I failed?' and 'What would people say about me for leaving a good secure job?' Looking back, it still amazes me how difficult it was for me to see the whole picture.

The value of the 30,000-foot bird's eye view, which I spoke about earlier, is that it allows you to see the whole picture. It removes you from the situation and allows you to see it for what it truly is, without emotional attachments. It wasn't until I had the conversation with my mum and she told me that, if I failed, I'd be in exactly the same situation as I was in now that I had the courage to make the leap.

Yet, it's difficult for us to remove ourselves from our

own story. To give an extreme example, I've seen the same thing happening with alcoholics and drug addicts. Their marriages fail; they lose their houses; some even end up in jail before they realise their addictions are not working for them. They live in this constant state of denial. Fortunately, most of our problems are less severe than drug addiction, but that doesn't make the recognition any easier. Take your job, for instance. Are you in denial about what you would really like to be doing? Worse yet, do you do what I did and tell everyone how happy and fulfilled you are when you're not? Are you living a lie?

I did exactly this when I was working sixteen hours a day right after my daughter was born. I was a full-blown workaholic and spent morning until night working on my 1:1 personal training business, mentoring other trainers who worked under me and growing an online business. I was obsessed with working and making more money. I didn't – or, more hurtful to admit, *wouldn't* – take time out of my day to meet my mum for coffee or read a story to my newborn daughter. I always worked and justified it with comments like 'I'm making great money', 'This is how I support my family' and 'This is what makes me successful'. My net worth determined my self-worth.

This came to a climax with one of those soul-destroying, life-forming moments. In 2016, I sat down with my mum on one of those rare occasions when I took a break. She had been complaining about her job, and her patience was at the end of its rope. She had spent over thirty years of her life working to support our family, so I told her to quit and I would hire her. My mum hated her job, and I was in the fortunate position to employ her, so I did. In that moment, I thought I had 'made it' and I was the best son on the planet.

Nevertheless, two months later, as I grew more and more stressed and withdrew even more from everyone around me, my mum sat me down one night at the kitchen table. I had been miserable, withdrawn and moody ever since I hired her (I was actually like this for several months prior, but she only noticed it now that she was working with me). I had been sleep-deprived, exhausted and self-medicating with work. The conversation with her was life-changing, but it hurt more than any ultramarathon or triathlon ever could. I had been giving myself a pat on the back for employing my mum for the past two months, but as she was working for me now, I made even less time for her. To add to that, as I was stressed out I took out my frustrations on her. As a side note, it still amazes me how we take out and project our own issues on the ones closest to us while hiding behind a mask in front of the rest of the world. We act like everything is okay, and we're nice and friendly to everyone, but as soon as we're behind closed doors, we take out our frustrations on the ones that love us most. If you have ever done this, change it today.

Anyway, I remember my mum sat me down on a cold October day and offered to quit her job with me and go back to work. I was shocked. She hated her last job, and I thought I was the best thing since sliced bread for hiring her. Yet, she thought my anger and withdrawal were aimed at her. The truth was she was just receiving all my projected issues because she was there. She was physically around me, so if I was having a bad day it was projected onto her.

Obviously, it was never intentional, but I lacked the self-awareness to realise that my mother didn't care if I earned minimum wage or millions. She valued the time with her son, not a wage packet from him every week. Earlier, I spoke about obstacles being the way, and my mother's offer to quit working for me was a turning point. It was the first time I realised that although my ladder was against the right wall, I was too focused on climbing that one single ladder at the expense of everything else.

That day, I convinced my mum not to quit, hired another person to cover all the outsourceable tasks and I reduced my own working hours. Now in 2019, I still meet my mum every week for lunch or coffee (it's non-negotiable) and the same applies to my daughter for our daddy–daughter days. I share the story because it's so easy to get caught up in denial and ignore the reality around you. My story was 'the more money I make, the more successful I am' and hiring my mum served as reinforcement for that idea. We all have blind spots, but it's up to us how to react when somebody points them out to us: 10% of life is what happens to you; 90% is how you react to it.

The truth is that your inner circle, whoever it may constitute, love you for who you are. They don't care if you earn more money, have better social status or possess the best physique on the planet. Yet, sometimes we make decisions that feel like they do. When you determine who will cry when you die and stop ignoring the reality around you and value the valuables, everything in your life will get better from that point forward.

Take action now

Take the time right now to make a list of what isn't working in your life. Ask yourself, 'What's not working right now?' 'Where is my ladder up against the wrong wall?' 'Are my actions mapping onto my ambition?' 'How can I improve the problem?' and 'What action do I need to take today?'

If you're good at removing yourself from any given situation and taking that 30,000-foot bird's eye view, then do it by yourself. I normally like to use resources, tools or people who help me see things from another viewpoint. If I have a problem in my business that needs to be solved, I look for books on the topic, then podcasts or blog posts, and finally seminars or consultations with experts to fill any gap in my knowledge. The key is to choose one action you can take and then do it. Then pause, make sure that action helped and then decide what you have to do next. Essentially, if your ladder is up against the right wall, you keep taking actions until you get the situation resolved. Once you have the end vision in mind, it's just about focusing on hitting that end goal.

11

Rewire Goal Setting

How to set goals

Goals and focusing on whatever target you are aiming at have been a thread flowing throughout this entire book. You cannot hit a target you can't see, and random actions will lead to random results; but, if you get very clear on whatever goal you set for yourself, the world will literally start to change in front of you. What you focus on is what will expand.

In 2001, a group of scientists in the Netherlands conducted an experiment to measure the effect of goals on perception.[1] You may be familiar with the term 'the law of attraction' – the New Age philosophy that if you believe in something hard enough, it will automatically come into your life. This experiment helps to explain

---

[1]   H Aarts, A Dijksterhuis and P De Vries (2001) 'On the Psychology of Drinking: Being thirsty and perpetually ready', *British Journal of Psychology*, 92, 631–642. www.goallab.nl/publications /documents/Aarts,%20Dijksterhuis,%20De%20Vries%20(2001)%20 -%20thirst%20and%20perceptual%20readiness.pdf

the cognitive neuroscience behind why the law of attraction may work.

The group of psychologists, led by Henk Aarts at Leiden University, began their trial the way so many scientists begin trials – by lying. Researchers often attempt to disguise a study's true purpose so that participants don't just play along or deliberately undermine the results. In this experiment, the researchers gathered eighty-four undergraduates for what Aarts described as a study on 'how well people can detect letters with their tongue under different taste conditions'. For example, can they detect the letter 'B' if the sweet was salty? It sounds ridiculous but what happened next was extremely interesting.

The study population was divided into two. One group got three Bisaldrops, a Dutch salty black liquorice sweet that makes you really thirsty, and each sweet was branded with a letter. Each person in that group had a minute to eat each candy and try to name the letter printed on it. The second group – the control group – received no candy at all; they were given instructions to trace three simple figures on paper, a form of busy work that had nothing to do with the experiment.

Afterwards, the researcher led the participants, one at a time, into a room he described as his office, to fill out a one-minute questionnaire on unrelated topics – 'What's your favourite activity to relax?' and similar questions. The questions had nothing to do with the aim of the study either. It was the room itself that was important. It looked like a standard academic office: a small space with a chair, desk, papers, books, pencils and a computer, among other things. Scattered about were several drink-related items, too – water bottles, a glass, cups, an empty soda can, a bottle lid, etc. After finishing the questionnaire, each participant sat in that office, by themselves, for four minutes.

The researcher then returned and brought the participants back to the lab for a surprise quiz. Each participant was given four minutes to write down as many objects from the office as they could remember.

By this time, the participants must have been wondering what on earth writing down the names of the objects had to do with detecting letters with their tongue, but they did what they were told. Some recalled only a single item and others half a dozen. There's nothing surprising there; it's likely that some people were daydreaming for those four minutes and others scanning the room. It was *what* they wrote down that the psychologists were interested in, and that was where a significant difference became clear.

The group that had been given the salty sweets remembered twice as many drink-related items as the control group. They were thirsty, and that influenced what they noticed in the office and remembered later, even if they weren't aware *why* they remembered those things.

If you've ever walked into a room and noticed some-body wearing a pair of shoes, a t-shirt or a dress that you wanted to buy, then you've experienced something similar. The experiment was a clever demonstration of a fairly straightforward principle of social psychology: Having a foremost goal in mind (in this case, a drink) tunes our perceptions to fulfilling it, and the tuning determines, to some extent, where we look and what we notice.

If you're on the lookout for a new car, you'll start noticing all the car ads on- or offline. More than likely, those ads were always there, but now that you're on the search for a new car, suddenly they all seem to appear right in front of you.

The researchers who undertook the study reported, 'The results suggest that basic needs and motives cause a heightened perceptual readiness to register environmental cues that are instrumental to satisfying our needs'. In other words, we tend to notice things that can help us move closer to our goal. They concluded, 'It can foster the reduction of thirst by helping us to detect a can of Coke, a glass of water or a bottle of beer that would go unnoticed under other circumstances'.[2]

This is likely a hardwired evolutionary strategy that kept us alive thousands of years ago, which, on the surface, sounds like common sense, right? Of course, we look for a drinking fountain or a glass of water when we're thirsty or a snack machine when hungry.

---

2   H Aarts, A Dijksterhuis and P De Vries (2001) 'On the Psychology of Drinking: Being thirsty and perpetually ready', *British Journal of Psychology*, 92, 631–642. www.goallab.nl/publications /documents/Aarts,%20Dijksterhuis,%20De%20Vries%20(2001)%20 -%20thirst%20and%20perceptual%20readiness.pdf

Nonetheless, keep in mind that the thirsty students in this study were more likely than the others to notice not just bottles of water or cans of soda but *anything* in the room that was drink related – a cup, a saucer, a bottle cap.

Whether they were aware of it or not, their thirst activated a mental network that scavenged the landscape for anything linked to liquid. This is why the law of attraction can actually work if you take the action steps that get you closer to your end goal.

Once you set a goal, you start to notice different things in your environment – things that were in front of you all along but you had previously tuned them out. Psychologists call this 'tuning perception', whereby we focus on all the things around us that can help move us closer to our goal.[3] This applies to quenching thirst or hunger but it also works for setting fitness-, relationship- or work-related goals. If you decide to get in shape, you would start noticing gyms everywhere. If you decide you're ready to get into a committed relationship, you would start noticing all the dating apps out there. If you decide to look for a new job, you would begin to see advertisements everywhere. It's tuned perception.

This is a familiar experience to all of us, but we tend to miss it. As soon as we decide to buy a certain brand

---

3   C Salahub and S Emrich (2016) 'Tuning Perception: Visual working memory biases the quality of visual awareness'. *Psychon Bull Rev*, Dec; 23(6): 1854–1859. www.ncbi.nlm.nih.gov/pubmed/27206649

of handbag or model of smartphone or style of jeans, we begin seeing that product far more often than we had before, in stores, online or while walking down the street.

I remember the first time this phenomenon occurred to me. I was fifteen years old, and I'd just bought my first pair of Adidas Predator football boots, which were standard issue and the best football boots you could get at the time. I wanted the pair in the style worn by my favourite footballers – the black, white and red shoes. I remember working for a month and a half to save for the boots, and the first time I wore them to a game, those boots were everywhere! I must have counted four or five pairs at that game alone. Not only that, over the next few weeks I started to notice the shoes in other, more exotic colours as well as different styles and designs. Within a month, I had a detailed mental map of a particular subculture: teenage footballers with Predator football boots in the West of Ireland – a subtle, intricate universe previously invisible to me.

This is why affirmations or writing your goals down is so important. You hone your tuned perception skills to identify things you may miss otherwise. If you're looking to lose body fat, then it helps to write that goal down regularly so that you can see it. Once you do, you're more likely to notice the great personal trainers, supportive books or online courses that can help you get there faster. The same goes for every single goal you set. Write it down, put it somewhere you can see regularly and keep an eye on the things you start to notice. I do this with every goal I set in all four of my quadrants.

Below is my step-by-step strategy for hitting any goal:

I. Write the goal down – it's all about visualisation

You can't hit a target you cannot see. As soon as you get clear on your goals for the four quadrants, write them down. If you want to lose weight, develop abs or drop three dress sizes, write that down. If you want to save £1,000 over the next twelve months, write that down. If you want to have a day every week just for you and your immediate family, write that down. If you want to start your own side-hustle business or sign up for an event that makes you feel more fulfilled, write that down. After that, you will start to see how tuned perception kicks in. Visualisation works if you put in the work. If you can see it in your mind; you can hold it in your hand, but the first step is writing it down. One of my mentors used to tell me, 'The only difference between a dream and a goal is writing it down'.

2. Write it as if you've done it already, then wait for reality to catch up

Write down your goals as if you have already achieved them. I had to deal with the 'imposter syndrome' for so long – that feeling that comes when you don't feel like you deserve what you got even after you hit the end goal. Even though I was helping people, that nagging voice would still pop up in my head with the thoughts, 'You don't know what you're talking about' or 'What do you know?' or 'Who will listen to you anyway?' My inoculation against this was writing my goals down as self-fulfilling prophecies, as if I had already accomplished them.

Before I wrote the first word of my first book *The Fitness Mindset*, I wrote down on my whiteboard 'I'm a best-selling author'. The book sold thousands of copies during its first week and remained in the bestseller list for over two months.

Now I didn't just wish for it to happen and sit on my sofa at home drinking tea. I started to write and edit the book as a best-selling author would. I was relentless with the editing process constantly asking, 'How can I word this better?' or 'Does this section really help people, and is it clear?' If the answer was no, the section was cut from the book or was rewritten. No waffle, no faff. If I wanted to be a best-selling author, I needed to write a book that helped and served thousands of people. Writing that goal as a self-fulfilling prophecy not only made me write more clearly and precisely, it also made me believe that it wasn't an unrealistic goal.

Every morning when I would sit down to write, I would see the goal 'I'm a best-selling author', and it got hammered into my subconscious that it had already happened. Now I was just waiting for reality to catch up.

Does it work with everything? No. I can't write, 'I'm going to play in the NBA this September' and expect it to come true, as I'm in my thirties, 5'8 and built like a hobbit. That goal, along with not being important to me, has many factors outside of my control.

Yet, as you saw earlier in this book, I used this exact process to become a professional fitness model, run six back-to-back marathons in the Sahara and run 230 km through the Arctic Circle. I intend to continue to do it going forward.

Write your goal down as if you've already achieved it and start making decisions as the person who's achieved it. Then, just wait for reality to catch up with you.

3. Put it somewhere you can see it – tuned perception

What you focus on is what will expand. Similar to writing down 'I'm a best-selling author' on the white-board in front of my work desk, I write down all my relevant goals somewhere I can see them regularly. My four quadrants are a constant fixture on my bedroom wall and allow me to stay focused on what it is I want to achieve. You saw the example of tuned perception from the Netherlands study above; now think about the compound effect of seeing your goal every morning when you wake up and every night before you go to bed. I guarantee if you take this single step, you will start noticing things you didn't see before. Putting down your goal in writing somewhere you can see it will prompt tuned perception to take over and do half the work.

These are my three tactics for goal setting. However, I've combined them with two other philosophies to give my strategy that extra edge. Combine all five together and you can hit any goal you set for yourself.

4. Always keep the end in mind – the power of focus

There is no big secret to goal setting: set the goal, take the action steps required, adjust course as needed, hit the end goal. Although that may appear pretty simple and straightforward, the application can be difficult.

If you've ever watched a soccer game, you know how this works. There are two goal posts, and each team tries to score in the opponent's goal post. Every tactic and every action step they take is to hit that end goal. They adjust how they do it based on feedback; if the opponent's right side of the team is strong, they attack from the left and try to score that way. They keep adjusting course until they hit the goal, but they always have the end goal in mind.

When you set a goal, always bear the end in mind. The reason I put down all my goals in writing some-where I can see them is because it allows me to stay focused, especially when life throws me a curveball.

When your routine is disrupted because of new work or family commitments, it's easy to skip a workout or not prioritise family time. That's how life is. It's not a linear path; it's up, down and sometimes sideways.

Keeping the end goal in mind, however, allows you to navigate around these obstacles as they occur.

If weight loss or improved fitness is your end goal, then you may have to get up an hour earlier next week to get your training session in. If getting up earlier is what you have to do, in order to avoid missing work or family commitments, then that's what you do. Remember, successful people do what they have to do whether they feel like it or not. Think about why you're trying to achieve the goal in the first place and stay focused on that. After that, it's just about breaking your goal down into smaller action steps.

5. Focus on small action steps – chunking

'There's only one way to eat an elephant. A
bite at a time.'
— Desmond Tutu

The biggest goals can be broken down into smaller component parts. When I worked as a math teacher, we used to call it 'chunking'. The most difficult math problems could be broken down into smaller parts and worked out in step-by-step processes.

Every single goal is exactly the same. When I decided to run six back-to-back marathons in the Sahara, I didn't focus on 230 km. I focused on being able to run 5 km, then 10 km, then 20 km, and so on. I worked off the 'pyramid of prioritisation' principle. There's no point worrying about six back-to-back marathons if I can't even run a single marathon, so I built up to running one and went from there.

You don't have to run through the Sahara or even complete a marathon, but every big goal you set for yourself in your personal life, professional life or financial life can be broken down into small action steps you need to take.

Keeping the end in mind by itself can sometimes be too daunting, as the goal may feel too big and unattainable. If you're like me, you may get what I call 'paralysis by analysis' – where you overthink the situation, become overwhelmed by the size of the end goal or what it will take to get there, and end up taking no steps at all.

Still, when you focus on 'controlling the controllable' and asking the question 'What action can I take today that moves me one step closer to this goal?' your focus will shift. Now you're no longer worrying about what's outside of your control – the future – and controlling what you can – the present. You're asking yourself, 'What can I do today?'

Always keep the end goal in mind. Every soccer team knows they want to score a goal, but focus on the small action steps: 'What side will we attack?' 'What action can we take right now?' Set a big goal and then break it down.

It is said that, 'The greater danger for most of us lies not in setting our aim too high and falling short, but in setting our aim too low and achieving the mark'.

Who or what is leading your life?

'Everyone thinks of changing the world, but no
one thinks of changing himself.'
— Leo Tolstoy

Here is yet another question for you to ask yourself:
'Who or what is leading your life or affecting the decisions you make?' Is it the approval of others? Pleasing
your mother or father? Others' expectations of you?
Maybe it's just proving yourself to yourself?

How you answer the question is pivotal to understanding what drives you, and it can give you back
control of the choices you make. If you're constantly
doing things to please your parents or look good in
front of your friends, that's not going to be enough
when times get tough – and they will get tough. Let's
face it: Change is hard, and becoming the best version
of yourself is difficult. If it were easy, everyone would
do it. Everyone would look the way they want to look,
feel the way they want to feel and have whatever they
want to have. I'm not saying it's easy to get the things
you want – the body, the job, the relationship. On
the contrary, it's very hard. It's hard to change your
thinking and put new action steps in place, and I can't
promise that it'll always be straightforward. But I can
promise one thing. When you decide to make new
decisions that map onto your ambition, your life will
get better and it *will* be worth it.

Owning the problems or issues in your life is never
easy. It's easier to blame other people. It's easier to

numb out with gossip, drugs or excessive consumption of entertainment. It's hard to own the part of yourself that you're unhappy with. It's hard to admit that you feel scared, insecure and uncomfortable. But as someone who has spent years trying to figure out why I was so mentally weak, I implore you to rewire that fear as a positive thing, as fuel for the fire and get comfortable with being uncomfortable.

When we build our lives around the things that are important to us and get our ladders up against the right wall in all four of our quadrants, every aspect of our lives can transform.

Right now, you are at a fork in the road in some area of your life – your health, your wealth, your love, your fulfilment or whatever you decide to split your focus on. Now and always, you have a choice to carry on as before or invent yourself anew. In *Meditations*, Marcus Aurelius said, 'The universe is change'.[4] When you differentiate a good change from a bad change, everything will open up before you.

Good changes get you closer to your end goal and bad changes move you further away from the end goal. If you're trying to lose weight or build some muscle, a good change may be joining a gym or starting a new workout regimen from home. A bad change is starting to go to a fast-food restaurant on your way from work every day.

---

4   *Meditations* by Marcus Aurelius, 161–180 AD. First translation in 1792 by Richard Graves.

As discussed earlier, our habits are what create our results. Therefore, it's up to you to consciously decide your habits and not allow them to mindlessly be thrown together or 'just happen'. It's true that you can't control your upbringing or genetics. You may have been born into poverty or a broken home, or be short, small or genetically inclined to gain weight. Cool, own that. You can't choose the cards you are dealt but sure as hell can choose how to play the hand.

Your handwriting is bad, so you're stupid!

I did terribly in school all throughout my teenage years. My handwriting was (and still is) nearly illegible to everybody but me. This meant I failed or only just passed every test or exam throughout high school. The fact that I could play sports helped me with some teachers, but others regularly called me everything from 'stupid' and 'dumb' to an 'idiot'. I couldn't write legibly, so, in their eyes, that was what I was.

However, born out of this was an ability to verbally articulate my words in a very comprehensive way. True, I wasn't able to write my ideas down on paper, but if given the chance to speak, I could use my verbal skills to break down even the most complicated of ideas, especially if it was related to subjects I enjoyed – food science and biology (my two best subjects). Having worked as a primary school teacher for several years, I now realise that I had an undiagnosed form of dysgraphia, but at the time, I was unaware of it. In the 90s, you were just labelled 'stupid' or 'slow' if you couldn't read or write well.

I wanted to share this anecdote for two reasons. First, out of every perceived setback is an opportunity if you choose to see it. The reason it can be hard to recognise it is that it normally doesn't become noticeable until after the fact. As Apple founder Steve Jobs said, 'The dots generally don't connect going forward; they only connect looking backwards, but you have to trust that the dots will connect in the future'.[5]

Richard Branson, the billionaire owner of Virgin, was dyslexic and failed most of his high school classes, but he used this to his advantage to see things from an outside-of-the-box perspective, and it led him to become one of the most successful entrepreneurs of all time. Every potential setback may seem bad at the time, but if you keep your mind open, you'll see an opportunity present itself from within it.

The second reason is that I went on to have a pretty successful career in academia. I spent five years in university and got two degrees (both with honours) and several other certificates and accreditations in sports nutrition, physical health and fitness training. At university, I was allowed to use a keyboard to type my assignments instead of writing, and I started to get top grades. The confidence that came from securing

---

5   Taken from Steve Jobs' 2005 Stanford University, CA
     Commencement speech. https://news.stanford.edu/2005/06/14
     /jobs-061505/

top grades made me question all the other self-limiting beliefs I held when it came to education. I had barely scraped through high school and just about scored enough to get into university, and now I was excelling.

I spent the next ten years learning more than I did through all of my previous schooling combined. The self-limiting story that I wasn't smart was now blown right open. With that, I added more legs to my confidence table.

That experience allowed me to become so proficient at articulating ideas in writing that it led to the writing of my first best-selling book, *The Fitness Mindset*, and the book you're currently reading.

Regardless of where you grew up or what life threw at you, success is about how you respond to that. See every obstacle as an opportunity to be better, to be stronger, to be tougher, and you'll never come up against an obstacle again. You'll welcome the challenge.

12

Rewire Your Mental Health

Rewiring your mindset consists of several different elements. So far, we have discussed everything from self-doubt and confidence to the compound effect and habits. There are two final pieces to the jigsaw puzzle for becoming the best version of yourself. One is your physical health, which is discussed in Chapter Thirteen, but before we come to that, I want to discuss the side of health that normally plays second fiddle to physical health, and that's our mental health. The undercurrent of mental health has flowed through this entire book but right now we are going to jump head first into it. The opening chapter of this book is titled 'Rewire Your Happiness', and some people think the opposite of happiness is sadness. For me, it's a little bit stronger than that. Sadness is one step removed from what I consider the bedrock of poor mental health, and that's misery.

Three things making you miserable that you never even thought of

As I mentioned earlier in the book, there are three types of knowing – the things you know, the things you don't know, and the things you don't know that you don't know.

The things you don't know that you don't know is where most of the pain in life originates. If you know how to do something or what you need to do, it's just about finding ways to be mentally stronger, cultivating the discipline and then mapping your actions onto your ambition.

If you don't know something, you at least know that there's a gap in your knowledge. To bridge that gap, you can read a book on the topic, listen to a podcast, do a course or attend a seminar. There are countless ways to find the information you need.

The things you don't know that you don't know are really difficult to handle because when you don't know you don't know something it can make you miserable (like in the examples in this chapter). Also, because of their subtlety, in most cases, they can make you wilfully blind to what's really making you unhappy. An unknown unknown masks itself with a positive feedback loop of: 'I do this thing. I feel better. Then I feel bad again. I do the thing again. I feel better again' and the cycle continues.

The examples below all fall into that trap. They normally move us away from pain, even if it's just a temporary escape from the painful reality of feeling unfulfillment or restlessness at the moment. As human beings, we constantly move away from pain and towards pleasure, but if you ever witness a drug addict hooked on heroin or crystal meth, you'll realise always and consistently seeking pleasure isn't a good thing.

Identifying the different types of pleasure you get is more important than simply seeking pleasure. The pleasure that comes from setting a goal and achieving it compared to the pleasure that comes from eating a full tub of ice cream that you hadn't planned on eating are very different. One gives you increased self-worth and confidence, and the other does the opposite.

Identifying the differences between the pleasures that are serving you and the ones that are making you weaker can be a massive indicator of how happy you'll feel going forward. The following examples are just some scenarios I've experienced and ironed out over the years. I'll share them in case they're the same for you or work as the triggers to unsupportive traits or habits you have.

1. Gossiping and talking about other people

This habit is one of the hardest to break, as it's hard-wired in our DNA. We're evolved social creatures, and in ancient times, being able to communicate and use language was one of the main reasons Homo sapiens climbed to the top of the food chain.

In the past, we lived in small hunter-gatherer groups built upon a social hierarchy. Historically, we lived in small groups or tribes of 50–100 people. The reason we could function so well as a society was our ability to use our language skills not only to hunt but also to keep track of other people in our tribe. Around 20,000 years ago, there were no smart devices or electronics, so it's likely that hunter-gatherers congregated around an open fire at night and talked about the things that happened during the day alongside the coming and going of others. Again, in a small group of 50–100 people, knowing who you could trust, who was a good hunter or who was strong or quick could literally make the difference between life and death. This is where evolutionary psychologists believe gossip originally developed.[1]

Similar to a lot of other emotional and primitive hardwiring I discussed earlier, our emotional limbic system takes over our inability to separate the rational from the emotional. Gossip is another one of those lower levels of thinking.

Now don't get me wrong. Gossiping and talking about other people can serve a tremendous purpose, and this is where your inner circle comes in. For example, the more information I have about my daughter's friends – what they're like, their previous actions (good or bad) – the better advice I can generally offer when asked about a problem or opportunity she has. But knowing about Jane or Joe down the street doesn't help my life in any way. If Jane is cheating on Joe or Joe is

---

[1]   D Buss (1998) *Evolutionary Psychology: The new science of the mind.* London: Taylor & Francis.

swindling money from his boss, neither would work great as a partner or employee, but my judgement about them doesn't move my life forward in any way.

The real trap for me in such a situation is what I call 'superiority bias'. You hear about people doing worse than you, and it makes you feel a little better about your own life, especially if you feel that person is of a higher social status than you. We evolved through complex hierarchical social structures that are mostly built upon zero-sum thinking. For one person to climb, it generally means another person had to fall. This is one of the reasons you may feel an endorphin rush when your boss is chewing out the work colleague above you, as you subconsciously feel it moves you ahead in the pecking order.

The same thing happens in the case of Joe and Jane. You may be miserable in your job, but seeing Joe's wife cheat on him makes you feel a little better about your life. I know because I did this for years. I had this horrible habit of comparing myself to the people who were perceived to be doing better than me in my given success metric at the time – better looking, bigger or leaner, wealthier, etc.

Because of the comparison, it always felt good when something 'bad' would happen to one of those people. This was never conscious, and I would never have admitted it, even if you pushed me for a comment, but it felt good inside. That's why it is so dangerous. That way of thinking kills you from the inside out.

I can pinpoint several reasons why I didn't achieve

any of my goals during the early part of my adult life, but comparing myself with others was probably the single biggest contributor. Unfortunately, it took me years to realise that comparison was the symptom, not the disease. The seed of the disease grew from the vicious habit of gossiping – my constant focus on other people, knowing what they were doing and knowing more about them than about myself!

Once, at a business conference, I met a woman in her early to mid-thirties, and we conversed back and forth. During the break, she told me how much she hated her boss and was only at the conference because he had made her attend it. She also told me about how she thought he was having an affair with his secretary and how much his wife gave out about him when she came to the office. In between stories of her boss, she also confided in me that her dream was to write a children's book someday. Obviously, as someone who makes a living by directly helping people achieve their goals, I probed her about her writing plans. She had a lot of excuses – no time, no money, no audience, etc. She offered all the usual self-sabotaging stories that derail us before we even get started, but her face did light up when she talked about it.

I tried to offer some input but quickly realised that it wasn't welcome, so I listened for another minute or two before turning back to my conference notepad. During this time, a cover band playing in between the keynote speakers played a hit song from some top rock band. I started bobbing my head, and the woman asked, 'You like this song?' I replied, 'Yeah, it's great. I don't know the name, though'. In an exaggerated tone, she responded, 'How do you not know the name of this song. It was #1 in the charts for seven weeks. It was always on the radio. The lead singer is going out with... ' and this dialogue went on for about two minutes straight.

It was at that moment I realised why she had not achieved any of her own dreams. All her thinking was about others! Remember, what you focus is on is what will expand. She knew about her boss's personal life. She knew who was going out with whom. She knew how many weeks the song had been #1 in the charts. Yet, she couldn't answer the question of what made her happy or give any real reason for why she wasn't writing her book.

She had numbed herself by consuming all the external world's gossip. I'm sure the dislike she felt for her boss was eased by the knowledge of his infidelity, but do you think that helped her write that book? No. I'm sure keeping the facts about the top songs probably gave her a sense of purpose or superiority bias when she could spout the numbers to someone who didn't have that knowledge, but did that make her happy long term? Probably not.

Unfortunately, this encounter struck me so much because I had done the exact thing in my early adult life. While working full time as a primary school teacher, I dreamt of something more. I wanted to work in fitness. I wanted to write books. I wanted to push my physical limits. But I was too afraid, afraid of failure: What would happen if I failed? What would people say?

Maybe I was also afraid of success. What if I got what I wanted, and I couldn't handle it? What if I got what I wanted and realised it wasn't what I truly wanted all along? What would I do then?

All lower-level thinking, but it consumed my thoughts throughout my twenties. Those thoughts are what I focused on, so they are what expanded.

This was the first encounter I'd had where someone else's words and actions mirrored back a person I once was. That was why it struck me so much. It also planted the seed for this section of the book as it made me ponder why we, as people, gossip. Why do we talk about others? Why do we feel good if they fail? Why do we need to know everything about them? The answer I got back was simple: It's easy to do.

It's easy to talk about others because their problems make us feel better about our lives. It's easy to feel good when they fail, as it serves as false reassurance that we don't really need to step up our game.

It's easy to learn mundane facts, as it makes us feel superior or smart when we regurgitate them back at people. For example, when I was twenty-four I could tell you every single fact about every single player on the football team I supported – I knew who played in the reserves that week, and who had the most assists or complete passes in last week's game. But I couldn't tell you what made me happy, what made me fulfilled. All

I knew was that I would feel confident and comfortable around other football fans because I had information I thought was valuable, but it was only needless information wrapped around my inner insecurity.

It's worth asking yourself the question, 'How much useless information am I storing in my head?' Think of your mind as a storage box. You can only keep so much in there. If you fill it with all that useless information about celebrities, sports teams or neighbourhood gossip, then you can't use that space to store information about the things that make you happy, put you into a positive state and make you feel fulfilled. I'm not saying not to partake in gossip or watch your favourite sport or follow your favourite celebrities at all. I'm just saying that you can't fill your storage box with such information and expect to fit in the other things that are important to you as well.

This brings me back to the 80:20 Pareto distribution mentioned earlier. Spend 80% of your time talking with people in your inner circle, consuming information that moves your life forward and asking questions about what makes you happy. Use the other 20% to do whatever you want – watching your sports team, gossiping with your friends or whatever thing you enjoy doing the most.

I've been on the flipside of this distribution where 80% of my time was spent on mindless and needless things and the end of the road was a lack of fulfilment and overwhelming restlessness.

Thoreau said, 'The mass of men live lives of quiet desperation'.[2] If you don't know where you currently are, it's impossible to know where you need to go, so first identify your starting point and where you are on that 80:20 spectrum, then decide if it needs to be changed.

I made the decision to not spend my time on mindless and needless things in my mid-twenties and never looked back. I have mentors who didn't learn the lesson until their forties, and others much later. It's never too late to make a change, but you have to get real with your starting point as you may not be happy with your answer.

That's okay. Lean into that discomfort and fear. If something isn't big enough to challenge you, then it isn't big enough to change you anyway. If it's big and scary to think about, good, it should be! It should be hard. Embrace that, because on the other side of fear is the person you want to be. If you can get conformable with discomfort and fear, I am confident your life will continue on an upward spiral from this point onwards.

When I left that conference, I had actually asked the woman her name and told her I would come to her first book signing when she finally published her book. I'm still waiting, but I've kept the name for safe keeping, just in case.

---

2   H D Thoreau (1854) *Walden, or, Life in the Woods.* Boston: Ticknor and Fields.

2. Telling white lies

I spoke about lying earlier, but white lies such as, 'Yes, you look great in that dress/jeans/T-shirt,' when you, in fact, believe the opposite, are the really dangerous ones as they're small and can pass by you pretty much undetected. White lies come down to handling the small things well. Tell me how you handle the small things and I'll tell you how you'll handle the big things.

3. Marrying your opinion to your self-worth

Negative comments aimed at our direction are just a part of life. Although we choose the emotions we attach to those words, it's inevitable that, sooner or later, we are going to come across people who hold a different opinion from us or disagree with what we believe.

It took me several years to disconnect my opinion from my self-worth. My inner need to belong to a group was palpable from my actions. I would change the way I spoke, alter my clothing and change my opinions just to try and belong. An old proverb states, 'We are too soon old and too late wise', and I spent most of my teenage years and early twenties trying to 'fit in'.

Ironically, it wasn't until I started to go down a different path in my mid-twenties that I started to find the people who I connected with the most, many of whom have become integral parts of my inner circle.

Still, there were some lingering bad habits that I had formed over these years that still caused me stress and anxiety. Those habits were mostly born from insecurity, and my extreme attachment to my ideas and opinions made me miserable for years. I struggled to deal with negative comments and took every slight personally. Then I learned that, for the most part, people don't generally attack you as a person. In some cases, they do; but, in most cases, they tend to attack your ideas or opinions. That one reframe allowed me to finally see the figurative forest from the trees.

When you learn to separate your opinion about things from your self-worth and who you are as a person, you tend to not take 'negative' comments so badly. As I mentioned earlier, you interject perspective into everything. If you have an ideology or belief system that is so strongly attached to who you are as a person, you will do everything in your power to protect or defend it, usually feeling miserable and closed off in the process.

You may identify with a fitness person, bodybuilder, runner, or identify as vegan or vegetarian, or be Christian, Jewish, Buddhist or Muslim, but that doesn't mean that's all you are. Just because somebody else holds a different belief system doesn't make either of you right or wrong. They're just opinions. Beliefs are just opinions that have been reinforced over and over again.

Yet, we attach ourselves so strongly to whatever belief system we hold and feel challenged if someone questions it. Other people can have different beliefs from you. That doesn't make them bad people. It just means they see the world from a different viewpoint.

We are tribal by nature, and we like it when we're around other people who believe the same thing we do. If you're religious, you may enjoy being around other religious people. If you support a certain sports team, you may identify with and prefer people who support the same team. My grandmother always told me, 'Birds of a feather flock together', and it's hardwired in our DNA to gravitate towards people who have similar beliefs or values to our own.

Growing up, I gravitated towards people who have similar beliefs or values to mine and hung around with other sports people. When I went into business, I did the same and identified with more than one tribe within the fitness community. Initially, I was a part of the bodybuilding community. Then, I adopted the CrossFit culture. Next, I followed a Paleolithic diet and swore that carbohydrate cycling was the best thing since sliced bread (no pun intended).

None of the beliefs I held at the time were really true, but I felt comfort in finding others who felt the same way as I did and felt attacked by anyone who held a different belief system from me. I would learn later in life that, 'It is a mark of an educated mind to be able to entertain a thought without accepting it'.

Nowadays, I generally don't feel I deserve to have an opinion on something unless I can argue the opposite side better than the people who hold that opinion. I love the apocryphal story of Socrates and his ability to distance himself from his best-loved ideas. His reputation as a philosopher – 'a lover of wisdom' – spread all over Athens and beyond. When told that the Oracle of Delphi had revealed to one of his friends that Socrates was the wisest man in Athens, he responded not by boasting or celebrating, but by trying to prove the Oracle wrong.

Socrates then decided he would try and find out if anyone knew what was truly worthwhile in life, as anyone who knew that would surely be wiser than him. He set about questioning everyone he could find, but no one could give him a satisfactory answer. Instead, they all pretended to know something they clearly did not. They were very educated in their specialisations and circles of competence (if they worked in science, they had deep knowledge in that area, for example), but once they went outside of that to give an opinion on politics, sports or some other field, they regurgitated some surface knowledge and acted like they knew more.

Finally, Socrates realised the Oracle must be right after all. He was the wisest man in Athens because he alone was prepared to admit his own ignorance rather than pretend to know something he did not. One of the most famous quotes attributed to him is: 'All I know is that I know nothing' – words I come back to any time I think I'm an expert at something.

How often have you offered an opinion on something that you don't really know anything about? Or how often have you talked to somebody who is clearly repeating some random sound bite that they read or heard?

There is nothing wrong with *not* having an opinion on something. If you don't have an interest in politics, sports or religion, then you don't need an opinion on it. If you're afraid people will think you're not intelligent or not well informed, then that's a sign of your own insecurity. That's a reflection of you, not them. Own that. If you can practice not having an opinion on every little thing, then it's good practice to disconnect from the opinions you do have so that you don't get so easily offended or anxious if challenged.

The reason I put so much emphasis on managing your opinions is once you realise that's all that they are, you understand any words or comments aimed at your direction are the same. They're opinions and perspectives, not truths or facts. This is the first step when learning to deal with any negative comment.

Once I started to do this, a lot of my internal stress and anxiety went away, and my bad habit of self-sabotage largely stopped as a result. I didn't feel the need to consistently fight with people who held an opposite opinion than that of my own.

This may sound trivial and your thought may be, 'I don't do that. I don't fight other people.' But think about any time you felt self-righteous over somebody else – maybe they eat food you know is bad for them or enjoy a movie you hate. These are examples of the small ways in which we let our opinions take hold and that becomes the habit that gets reinforced.

We grow attached to them and the confirmation bias kicks in, leading us to consume information or surround ourselves with people who further support our opinion and ignore any disconfirming evidence. This is what happened in Nazi Germany and Stalin's Russia. It's exactly how propaganda works. If you get told something often enough with people constantly reinforcing the idea, you start to believe it. That goes for every thought that enters your mind, and what you focus on is what expands. If you focus on all those opinions that you hold, then those opinions become beliefs. If you're not careful, they evolve into ideologies, and once they get to that level, it's very difficult to change them.

Over the years, the way I've tried to overcome this tendency is by going into every conversation assuming that the other person knows something I don't. Every conversation is an opportunity to learn something new. Sometimes, you realise pretty quickly that the conversation isn't going anywhere and cut it short, but other times, you get a unique opportunity to learn something you may not have thought of previously. The next time somebody disagrees with you, don't get angry, annoyed or defensive; instead, use it as an opportunity to learn something new. If you still disagree, realise that the other person is attacking or disagrees with your opinion, not you as a person. Your opinion and your character are not the same thing. Don't marry your opinion to your self-worth and your mental health will improve.

Comparing yourself to others

'Comparison is the thief of joy.'
— Theodore Roosevelt

Have you ever been having a pretty good day – everything is going well; you're happy with the way you look and the way your life is going right now – only to suddenly see something on social media or someone who looks like they have it better than you? With it, your mood drops.

It has happened to all of us in some area of our life. One moment, we are happy that we did our workout for the day. The next moment, we see someone who is leaner, bigger or skinnier, and suddenly our workout seems pointless. The negative self-talk of, 'Why don't I look like that?' or some variation of those words intrudes your mind. Or we study hard and do well in a test or an exam, only to learn a friend has done better than us. Again, the words, 'You're not as smart as them' – or, worse, 'Why do I even bother?' – pop into your head.

As I discussed earlier in the book with regard to gossip, such comparisons to other people served as an evolutionary benefit. If you saw somebody who was doing better than you, it allowed you to up your own game. The better you did, the more likely you were to climb the social hierarchy and inevitably pass on your genes. The people who had this innate ability did exactly this and they are our direct ancestors. Comparison is hardwired in our DNA, and although it may have served a great purpose to early Homo sapiens, nowadays it just makes us miserable!

Do you even care about tennis?

My incessant need to compare myself with people made me unhappy for so long. However, as I kept digging deeper into why I had this tendency, I realised something quite peculiar but glaringly obvious. I only compared myself against people who I saw as direct or indirect rivals in some way.

When you think about it, it's funny because we only compare ourselves to people who are similar to us or have similar values. I never once compared myself to the tennis professionals Roger Federer or Rafael Nadal because I never played tennis. If a work colleague did great in a tennis tournament, I would be genuinely happy for them most of the time. That particular achievement never served as a threat to my ego or what I perceived as a threat to my social status or position in that particular hierarchy. I don't play tennis, so people excelling in the area don't have any impact on my self-worth.

On the other hand, if it were somebody doing well in football or, later in my life, bodybuilding, instantly my 'comparison radar' would go into full swing. One of my mentors used to always tell me that, 'People want to see you do well, just not as well as them', and that's how I used to feel.

Instead of rewiring the way I saw it and using it as

fuel for my own fire (something I try and do now), I would be consumed by jealousy or envy at best and be despondent or depressed at worst. It pains me to admit how crippling these comparisons were but the seed of overcoming them was born from this despondency. As Carl Jung said, 'Your branches can't reach to heaven if your roots don't go down to hell'.[3]

In this book, I've mentioned countless times the importance of changing the way you see things and how your habits and what you do every day are what define you. For years, I would compare myself with people who were doing better than me, and it always affected me negatively. It wasn't until I got to the root of the insecurity (a lack of confidence) and realised it wasn't helping me to see things this way that I was able to change the way I saw things. I had to take responsibility for it and own it before I could change it.

The reason I use tennis as an example is that we all have our version of 'football' and 'tennis'. We have things we value consciously or subconsciously that can threaten our self-worth – such as money, social status, physical appearance, fitness, sporting ability or business acumen. We all have things that, even though we are impressed by them, don't shift our emotions in any significant way – tennis, for me.

I was giving too much energy, emotion and attachment to the external things that were valuable to me

---

3   C G Jung (1959) *Aion: Researches into the Phenomenology of the Self: Collected works of C G Jung.* London: Routledge.

until I realised those things were just that: 'valuable to me'. Only once I recognised this and started to focus on the things that were truly valuable – my family, my impact on others, my inner circle of friends – did I feel the wave of comparison wash directly over me and past me.

I implemented several strategies to help me get to this point. We're all living through this human condition, and I don't know if my tendency to compare myself with others will ever truly leave me, but when I feel my 'monkey mind' taking over and trying to highjack my higher-level thinking, I use one (or all) of the strategies below. I hope they serve you as much as they serve me.

I.   Compare against yourself

Comparison isn't necessarily a bad thing; in fact; it can be supremely positive and beneficial if you use it correctly.

Comparing yourself to other people, especially those who you perceive to be ahead of you, is a recipe for misery. However, comparing yourself to where you once were is crucial for two reasons: 1) it gives you direct feedback on how well you are doing, and 2) it allows you to shift direction or change strategies if you're not improving.

Similar to directing a ship from point A to point B, it doesn't really matter how you get to the end. You may go backwards, forwards and sideways, but as long as you get from where you are to where you want to be, that's what is most important. Every time I see my head turning in another direction, I try and bring my focus back to my goals.

In this context, an analogy I like to use is that of driving a car on a highway. If you're driving your car and looking around at the other drivers, it's inevitable you're going to crash and will probably never reach your end destination. Ironically, if you focus on driving your own car or 'running your own race', you normally end up passing most of the other drivers who are too busy looking around them.

Success leaves clues. If you are getting closer to the end goal, then keep doing what you're doing. If you're moving further away from the end goal, then something has to change. It's as simple as that.

2. Power of contrasting

On the days I'm not feeling quite as mentally strong, and my own progress seems minimal (we all have these days, by the way), I contrast my current situation to where I have been in the past. If I ever worry about money or an investment opportunity, I close my eyes and remember the time I had to go through the back of my sofa for money for a bus ride. I use the contrast to snap me back into a more grateful mindset. If I feel a bit flabby and soft from eating too much over the past few days, I think about when I ran out of food and was starving in the Sahara. Instantly, that makes me grateful for the extra food I've been able to eat over the last few days. If I get overwhelmed from too many speaking or work-related requests, I remember the time I was working two jobs with the hope that I'd 'make it' someday. These contrasts allow me to shift my mindset and change my state. Once your emotional state changes, your focus shifts and you start giving energy back to the things that are important.

3. Gratitude anchors

This is a simple idea but takes quite a bit of practice. Every time I feel low about some perceived 'lack', 'scarcity' or negative self-talk – I'm not smart enough, not wealthy enough, not big or strong enough – I think about three things I'm grateful for. Normally, it's small things like bringing my daughter to a movie or the playground, having coffee with my mum or getting to do my workout, but it's a simple mindset shift technique that gets me from a negative state to a positive one. I also do a 'gratitude journal' every morning where I take about two minutes to write down things that I'm grateful for. Over the years, I've noticed that this has subconsciously rewired my brain to notice the positive things in my life, and it's a tactic I still use.

4. Negative visualisation

When the gratitude anchors don't work, negative visualisation is the ace up my sleeve that normally shifts my state. I've spoken about negative visualisation earlier in the book, but this is the ultimate tactic I use when all else fails.

If I find I'm worrying about silly things – or, worse, things outside of my control (those I can't affect even if I wanted to) – then I close my eyes and think about losing the things I love most.

It's funny because what I visualise is not usually the thing I'm currently worrying about. If I'm worried about my appearance, that's not generally what comes to my mind during negative visualisation. If I'm worried about finances, again, it's rarely what appears when I close my eyes. It's normally a picture of my daughter terminally ill in the hospital or my mum in a car crash. Once you have identified the valuable things in your life, the things you can't put a price on, you picture those things being taken away from you, and it'll make everything else pale in comparison.

As I said earlier, this technique is the ace up my sleeve, and I only use it when I have to, but it generally shifts my focus instantly and removes all that nagging mental chatter or 'monkey mind' talk that comes with the routines of life. Use it as needed.

13

Rewire Your Lifestyle – Nutrition, Training and Sleep

Giving from an empty cup

The first twelve chapters of this book talk about rewiring your mindset. This chapter is focused more on rewiring your 'health-set'. Your 'health-set' is the things you do every day that improve your physical health. True, you may want to lose weight, get leaner, become stronger or build more muscle, but that's only your primary fitness goal so long as your health is in order.

My grandmother used to tell me, 'When you have your health, you have many goals. When you are sick, you only have one – to get better'. Prioritising your 'health-set' is important because, without it, nothing else matters. If you're lying in a hospital bed in pain, you don't care about work commitments or how low your body fat is; instead, you just want to find a way to alleviate the pain.

If you're at that point and reading this book, I hope some of the mindset rewiring sections in the earlier chapters have supported you thus far. That said, if you're reading this book and you're still in good health, then I implore you to adopt the Benjamin Franklin philosophy: 'An ounce of prevention is worth a pound of cure'. Don't wait for your health to decline before you worry about improving it. Take control of it now. If you haven't done it up until this point, that's fine. Own it. Now is the time to change it.

Nutrition, training and sleep have served as the anchors for my 'health-set' for the past ten years. As mentioned in earlier chapters, there have been times when they've been out of balance and other occasions when I couldn't prioritise them, but I always come to the same three anchors. If you've ever been on a ship, anchors are what sailors use to keep it in one specific location, to keep it 'grounded'. Nutrition, training and sleep are the anchors that can keep your life grounded. They help to keep it where you want to it to be.

Eating well, exercising consistently and monitoring my sleep serve all my greater goals. I'm a better father, friend and son when I am well rested. I'm able to serve and help more people because my energy levels are higher after morning workouts. I'm able to be more productive and concentrate better during the day because of the nutritious food I eat. *Looking after yourself first is not selfish; it's practical.* You can't be the best version of yourself for those around you if you're not the best version of yourself. Period. If you've ever been on an aeroplane, you may be familiar with the safety instructions they announce at the beginning of each flight. Can you remember what they tell you to do in case of an emergency? If the oxygen mask falls down, they tell you to put on your own mask first and then help small children, the elderly and other passengers. Flight attendants know you can't help anybody else if you don't look after yourself first.

I always think of it like trying to give from an empty cup. I regularly picture myself as a cup of water. If that cup is empty because I'm too unhealthy or fatigued, then I can't give anything from it. However, if I take care of myself, look after my health, physical body and energy levels, then that cup overflows. There's so much in it. It's easy to give it out. That's why looking after yourself first is not selfish; it's practical.

As you've read in earlier chapters, I've made the mistake myself in the past and resisted the ownership of this issue in particular, but once I took responsibility for it I took back control and was able to put the necessary changes in place.

Physical health anchors

The final piece of the puzzle is your physical health. It's true that you can rewire your mindset, not do anything with your physical health and still reap all the benefits of a better life. Yet, from my experience, I like to see it all interconnected.

The better you physically feel, the better you tend

to feel mentally and vice versa. Nutrition, training and sleep are the foundation anchors upon which physical health are built. This particular chapter may be daunting based on your background. If you've eaten well and worked out most of your life, you'll take the suggestions on board easily enough, and if you've never done anything physical in your life, you may have a mental barrier about their application, especially the nutrition section.

Fitness and nutrition are my specialisations, so I've covered these in significant detail in my first book, *The Fitness Mindset*, but here are some tips and tricks to rewire your lifestyle so that you have more energy and feel physically better every single day.

Nutrition

The saying 'You are what you eat' is very applicable when it comes to having more energy and feeling physically better. Regardless of whether your goal is weight loss, muscle building or just building a leaner and fitter physique, the foundation of energy is the food you eat. If you have a low-quality diet composed of fast and processed food, then your body is going to have low-quality energy. Combine this with too many calories and you'll start to see extra pounds creeping up over the coming months. Remember our example in the chapter on 'The Compound Effect'?

The truth is there are many incredible diets out there

and lots of 'not so incredible' diets – the key is finding the one sustainable for you. I wrote in my first book that the best diet is 'the one that includes foods that you enjoy, fits into your lifestyle and schedule and is in alignment with your end goal', and I don't think that philosophy will ever change as it's 100% adoptable by every single person.

Ice cream and chocolate may be foods that you enjoy and fit into your lifestyle and schedule, but if your goal is to lose weight, then it's probably worth reconsidering a diet based on them as an option. The same is true for eating salad and broccoli at every meal. The low calories may help you to lose weight and may even fit into your lifestyle and schedule, but I don't think I've ever met a person who enjoyed eating salad and broccoli for every single meal of every single day.

Again, the danger is in the dosage, and one serving of ice cream is not going to make you fat, the same way one salad at lunchtime isn't going to make you lean and skinny. It's what you consistently do every day that's important. The key is to focus on the process, not just the outcome. If you are trying to lose weight, you need to reduce calories gradually while maintaining your energy levels so your workouts and your day-to-day existence don't suffer.

If you're trying to build muscle, you may need to increase your protein intake to help you repair from workouts. Experimenting with different food groups and diets is always going to be the best option as you can find what works best for you. Nevertheless, there are a few golden rules you can apply that will instantly help with your energy levels and physical health.

1. Try and eat more whole foods

One of my golden rules is that if it has more than one or two ingredients on its label, I try and minimise it in my diet. An 80/20 split works well here. If 80% of your nutrition is whole food – single ingredients – then you're probably going to feel better throughout the day. Examples include the following:

- Fruit
- Vegetables
- Meat
- Fish
- Nuts
- Seeds
- Wholegrain foods such as oats, brown rice, sweet potato

These are just some of the options you can include. Experiment with what you enjoy the most.

The main foods to watch out for and minimise are highly processed refined sugar and fast food that is high in trans fatty acids. They are not only devoid of nutrients in comparison to the foods above but also loaded with extra calories that can make you fatter, as they're very easy to overeat, so keep an eye out for them.

2. The 70%-full rule

This one is pretty simple. Eat until you're 70% full. Eating until you can't move isn't generally the best idea. I take a primal approach to this one. I ask myself, 'If I had to run away from a predator right now, could I do it?' If I'm too full to move, I've overeaten and need to be more conscious of it in my next meal.

If I feel like I could still run, then that's when I stop eating. I'm fortunate I live in the developed Western world, not the African Savannah, and the chance of me coming face to face with something higher on the food chain is pretty slim. Though, this is the tactic I still use to this day, as eating until I'm completely full normally leaves me tired and lethargic.

Feel free to experiment with other variations that work better for you. I have a friend who uses the 'Could I have sex right now?' rule. When he's stuffed, the last thing he wants to do is have sex. So, to stop himself overeating at meals he deploys this tactic. I've never asked him what particular experience led him to the strategy, but I can only assume...

Of course, there are times when you have a family meal or you're on holidays, and by all means, enjoy that and eat to your heart's content. Just don't do it with every single meal of every single day. Not only do you risk consuming too many calories, which can add unwanted inches to your waistline, but also a 'dull' feeling comes with eating too much and makes it less likely you will do anything physical while your body digests all that food. Again, this is fine occasionally, just don't do it every day. You never know when that tiger – or in the case of my friend, that cougar – is lurking around the corner.

3. Eat more greens

Vegetables, especially leafy greens, are probably the most nutrient-dense foods that you can eat. They are loaded with micronutrients, vitamins and minerals that your body needs to function properly. Most are really low in calories, too, making them perfect as diet foods.

If you don't like vegetables, the secret is to start eating them gradually. Try adding a couple of florets of broccoli to your next meal or some chopped carrots into your soup. I never ate any vegetables until I was in my early twenties. As I learned about their health benefits, I started to add them to my diet gradually. First, I blended spinach in my fruit smoothie in the mornings. Then, I added broccoli to my favourite sweet potato soup. After that, I forced myself to eat a little bit at dinnertime until I started to build a taste for it.

Currently, my diet is mostly plant based. I enjoy eating that way, and I very rarely, if ever, get sick. This way of eating fuels my training sessions and provides the energy for my work commitments. There is no secret to eating for energy. Eat foods that have all the vitamins and minerals your body needs, and you'll feel better. It really is that simple.

Training

The second foundation anchor for improving your lifestyle is physical exercise. As mentioned earlier in the goal section, what you do is going to be dependent on your individual starting point. If you've never worked out in your life, then a twenty-minute walk around the block after work can serve as a great workout for you. If you're an advanced marathon runner, triathlete or bodybuilder, you're obviously going to do more than that. Nonetheless, here are some tips that nearly anyone can include to improve their physical fitness:

1. Train for your goals

Regardless of whether you're a beginner or an elite athlete, the principle here is the same. Although the tactics and the daily workouts may look completely different, the idea doesn't change – design your training programme around your specific goals.

If you want to lose weight, make sure your exercise programme includes lots of movement, high-intensity exercise or cardio in general. If you're trying to get bigger and stronger, then factor in several days of weight training each week.

2. Try some HIIT workouts

High Intensity Interval Training (HIIT) is exactly as it sounds – high intensity over intervals (ie, short periods of time). Again, it's goal dependent, but if you're looking to get fitter and leaner, it's hard to go wrong with this form of training. The beauty is you can do it almost anytime and anywhere. If you're in the gym, try the HIIT cardio from my first book *The Fitness Mindset*.

EXERCISE BIKE:

30:30 sprint

Description: On an exercise bike, set the resistance level to a point where it's hard to move the pedals but light enough to go quickly if you pedal hard. Next, set the timer for ten minutes. For the first thirty seconds over every minute, pedal at a normal speed. When the clock hits thirty seconds, go as fast as you physically can for the next thirty seconds. After thirty seconds are complete, relax and slow down again. Repeat this ten times.

The key to HIIT workouts is the intensity on the sprint. For some people, this works as their entire workout. For others, it's a great way to finish a session so you feel like you left it all behind you. You can also do the same regimen at home with bodyweight squats, push-ups and other exercises, so play around with it.

3. Add resistance training to your regimen

Again, if getting leaner, stronger or building muscle is your goal, consider adding some form of resistance or weight training to your programme. Resistance training is exactly as it sounds – creating extra resistance on your body so that you can get stronger or build more lean muscle tissue. You can do this through bodyweight resistance, machines or free weights. How much you actually do is based on your individual goals. I generally aim for three to five resistance sessions per week myself.

Sleep

Finally, we get to the last anchor for your 'health-set', and that is sleep. As someone who has been a notoriously poor sleeper most of his life, it's very simple for me to see how easily poor sleep quality can not only affect your mood and energy levels but also your overall life quality. Poor sleep can influence everything from your energy levels during training sessions to your willpower and ability to make better choices throughout the day.

I am not a sleep expert, and if this is an area of your life that you struggle with, I highly recommend checking out two books that will support you in becoming a better sleeper:

- *Why We Sleep* by Matthew Walker[1]
- *Sleep* by Nick Littlehales[2]

Both of these books go into significant detail, but here are two tips to get you started on improving your sleep quality.

---

1   M Walker (2017) *Why We Sleep*. New York: Scribner.
2   N Littlehales (2016) *Sleep*. London: Penguin Life.

1. Aim for seven to nine hours of sleep every night

Everybody has different sleep requirements, but most sleep researchers tend to agree that anything between seven and nine hours of quality sleep per night is ideal for most people.

Again, there is no 'one size fits all', so experiment with how much sleep you need. More isn't always better. When you've slept too much, you can wake up feeling the same as if you slept too little. I tend to find that I work well on seven and a half of hours of sleep. But if I'm training for an extreme challenge, this requirement goes up to nine hours per night. Test with different durations between that range and find what leaves you feeling the most recovered and refreshed.

2. Reduce overthinking by writing things down

In the past, I would spend an hour trying to fall asleep because my brain wouldn't stop rehashing the day's events. This was especially true in my early twenties, as every mistake I made in my life would replay over and over in my head at night-time.

Now, don't get me wrong. This kind of self-evaluation can be a very positive thing. It tells you exactly where you need to improve and gives you direct feedback on what you have to work on. If you dread going to work every single day, it may be time to consider a career change. If you're going to bed miserable because you're in a toxic relationship, then having some difficult conversations may be worthwhile. If you keep falling off your diet and can't stick to a workout regimen, maybe it's time to switch what you've been doing or hire a personal trainer for accountability.

Self-analysis is important, and the most successful people I speak with do it regularly. But when you're trying to wind down and fall asleep, it isn't the best time to think about all those things. If you're the kind of person who overthinks your day and replays mistakes over and over again in your head, my advice is to designate a specific time for doing this – either by yourself or with a friend or partner. Go over exactly what you did well and what you need to improve upon. Write it down somewhere, even if you never look at it again. There's a certain mental catharsis we can achieve from writing down the things that we need to work on. Then, we can leave them or come back to them in the future. I guarantee if it's playing over and over in your head, writing it down will make you feel a lot better and help you reduce your overthinking or anxiety after a stressful day.

14

Rewire the Ultimate Fear – You Are Going to Die!

> 'Remembering that you are going to die is the best way I know to avoid the trap of thinking you have something to lose.'[1]
>   — Steve Jobs

Disease of 'someday'

If we take on the challenge of self-improvement or self-invention, we will find ourselves walking down an unfamiliar road. Rather than being led by what has been important to us in the past, we will find ourselves working towards what we are committed to right now and working to that end goal. Success is doing what you have to do whether you feel like it or not and not waiting for 'someday' to happen.

Most people fall into the trap of thinking that they

---

[1]   Taken from Steve Jobs' 2005 Stanford University, CA
     Commencement speech. https://news.stanford.edu/2005/06/14
     /jobs-061505/

can work towards their dreams and they'll get around to doing it 'someday' or its kissing cousin 'when I have time'. The illusion of 'someday' or 'when I have time' is very persuasive, soothing and even tranquilising.

It feels good to convince ourselves that we're not putting it off. No, no, no, we just don't have time right now. It's the path of least resistance, and when you take that path, my God, does your life get difficult! As you've read countless times on this book journey, I did this with nearly every situation or scenario where I disguised fear as practicality. I wouldn't leave my safe teaching job because I told myself that 'someday' in the future, when things were a little more secure, that I would be able to start my own business.

I didn't step on a bodybuilding stage until 2014 because I told myself 'I don't have time for that right now'. It even took me five years to write my first book because I told myself that I could always come back to it 'someday'. To be honest, it actually only took about six months to write, but it took the other four and a half years to convince myself that I could do it.

Life doesn't fit into this 'someday' illusion: The daily news offers frequent reports of people dying in car accidents on their way to work. These people didn't wake up expecting that to happen. They were certain that it was just another day at work. Accepting the reality that you are not going to live forever is the first step towards living the life you want. I had that moment when I was walking down the street in East London and pictured myself attending my own funeral.

It made me realise that reality can be very rude in its surprises, and it doesn't care about how it intrudes on our hopes and dreams.

One of the things that would keep me awake at night was thinking about going to the grave with all my dreams inside of me, unrealised. I had dreams of the person I wanted to become, the books I wanted to write, and the life I wanted to create to serve others and ensure the world was a little bit better because I was here.

But if I died that night in East London, all those dreams would go to the grave with me. If you take nothing else from this book, tattoo this onto your brain: *Don't go to the grave with all your dreams inside of you!*

The cemetery is a scary place to walk through. As a child, it scared me because of the dead bodies. As an adult, it scares me because it's a constant reminder that the grave is where people's dreams go to die.

Own the fact that you're not going to be around forever. Control it by making the decisions that get your ladder against the right wall in all the important areas of your life. Change the way you see things from this moment onwards so you never become the person who goes to the grave with all their dreams inside of them.

I have one final tool in my toolkit to ensure that this never happens to you. I call it my '97-year-old rule'.

The 97-year-old rule

In Bronnie Ware's book *The Top Five Regrets Of The Dying*, the author documents her time spent tending to the needs of those on their deathbed. I came across this list of hers in late 2017 and it made me redefine some of the decisions I had been making up to that point. Before I continue, it's worth sharing her list:

REGRET 1: I wish I'd had the courage to live a life true to myself, not the life others expected of me.

REGRET 2: I wish I hadn't worked so hard.

REGRET 3: I wish I'd had the courage to express my feelings.

REGRET 4: I wish I had stayed in touch with my friends.

REGRET 5: I wish I had let myself be happier.[2]

Although these are the top five regrets according to the author's experience, they tend to hold true for most of us. Reading the list, a seed was planted for my 97-year-old rule.

The 97-year-old rule is the approach I take when it comes to making decisions on what I should do, who I should spend time with and where I should focus my attention. When making any life, business or family decisions, I ask myself, 'If I were on my death bed, what would my 97-year-old self regret more?'

This wider perspective always guides me in making

---

2   B Ware (2012) *The Top Five Regrets of the Dying*. London: Hay House UK.

better decisions. You may recall my example earlier in the book about coming home from the Sahara and, instead of going to work, I stayed at home with my daughter and watched Disney movies all day. That was the 97-year-old rule coming into full effect.

It is easy to get caught up in the day-to-day running of our lives, working to deadlines, following other people's calendars or even our own schedule, all the while missing the things that we would really regret if we were on our deathbed.

The next time you need to make any decision that affects you or the people closest to you, just ask yourself: 'What would my 97-year-old self regret more?' Once you've rewired your mindset around the ultimate fear, then going to your deathbed with no regrets is truly the way to live, in my opinion. In the Conclusion below, I mention that we can't stop the inevitable. We can't alter the final destination but we sure as hell can decide the journey we take to that end point. To paraphrase the great Roman philosopher Cicero: 'The best way to die, is to have lived a great life preceding it'.

None of us has reached the end of our journey yet, but arriving there with no regrets from this point forward is one of my major goals in life. Consistently asking, 'What would my 97-year-old self regret more?' has allowed me to overcome my own battle with fear, anxiety and lack of belief in myself over the years. Using the principles in this book, I built the confidence and self-discipline to go after the things that I wanted, and I encourage you to do the same. Once upon a time, running through the Sahara and the Arctic, having my daughter, writing books and public speaking all terrified me, but my 97-year-old self would have regretted not trying them out of fear. Silence that enemy between your two ears and go to your grave with no regrets.

Conclusion

If we could step back and somehow examine the train of our daily thoughts, we would realise how they tend to circle around the same anxieties, emotions and feelings, like a continuous loop. If left to your default thinking, even when we take a walk or have a conversation with someone, we generally remain connected to this inner monologue, only half listening and paying attention to what we see or hear. Upon occasion, however, certain events can trigger a different quality of thinking and feeling. Let us say we go on a trip to a foreign country that we have never visited before, outside our usual comfort zone. Suddenly our senses snap to life and everything we see and hear seems a little more vibrant. Life on autopilot is dull and bland. Life, where you are in full control of the way you think, is bright and colourful, and it is the greatest gift one can receive. All the same, we generally only appreciate gifts when we realise that they can be taken away from us. Therein lies the secret to happiness.

There is a saying that there are only two important days in your life, the day you were born and the day you realise you're going to die. For us humans, death is not only a source of fear but also of awkwardness. We are the only animal truly conscious of our impending mortality. In general, we have the power to think and reflect, and that's what makes us great. But in this particular case, if we don't rewire our mindset around the ultimate fear, then our thinking brings us nothing but misery. We either go through life never thinking about it, because of the discomfort it brings us, or if we do, all we see is the physical pain involved in dying, the separation from loved ones and the uncertainty of when such a moment might arrive. For every problem, there's a solution. The solution here is to take back ownership of everything in your life and realise that you're only getting one life. If you picture life as a journey, the end, by its design, is a part of every single journey. You can't control the ending but you can control the entire story that leads you to that point. Just remember this final quote that summarises the entire journey of this book.

'When writing the story of your own life, don't let somebody else hold the pen.'
— Harley Davidson

I hope this book has helped to support you on your journey. Please share it with your friends or family members who you feel will benefit from it as well.

Epilogue

It's 11.30pm on 20 February 2019. It's -38°C in the middle of the Arctic. I'm 70 km from the Arctic Circle line where I plan to finish the end of a gruelling 230km run through one of the harshest environments on the planet.

Like everything we do in life, it hurts and feels like a perpetual struggle, but I continue to put one foot in front of the other, and 70 km later I cross the finish line. The enemy between my two ears is dead. Now I implore you to do the same thing with your mindset. No more self-sabotage, no more seeing failure as a bad thing, no more waiting for 'somebody' to come. Today you start to own your life. Today you start to control and change it. You are going to die someday, so stop living like you've got forever. Take back control of your life, and from this day until your last: 'Don't let your biggest enemy live between your two ears!'

Acknowledgements

My gratitude goes out to all those who have passed through my life. All of you have contributed in some way to my journey and the substance of this book.

First, I want to thank my publisher Lucy McCarraher and Rethink Press. Without them, this book would not be possible.

My sister Karen, who has always been my second biggest fan in everything that I do. She has been one of my best friends and is one of the smartest people I've had the pleasure of knowing.

My father Gerry, who nurtured a work ethic and mental toughness that supports me to this day.

My friend Simon Halpin, who ran beside me through the Sahara and Arctic. His friendship and support have moulded my mindset to where it is today.

My best friend Paul Dermody who is the corner stone of my inner circle. He constantly makes me challenge my own best-loved beliefs and ideas which allows me to consistently grow as a person.

Finally, to whom this book is dedicated – my mum Rita and my daughter Holly. My mum and my daughter are the two closest people in my life. Without my mum, I wouldn't be on my current journey and have the gratitude mindset that I have; and without Holly, I wouldn't have my reason for doing what I do.

This book is dedicated to them, for without them, I would not be the man, son or father I am today. I love you both.

Thank you.

The Author

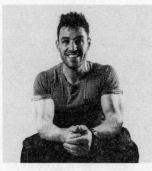

Brian is a motivational speaker, qualified personal trainer, sports nutritionist and business owner.

He is the best-selling author of the book *The Fitness Mindset* and currently travels the world as a professional speaker. He also hosts the #1 podcast: The Brian Keane Podcast.

Brian is a former primary school teacher turned fitness entrepreneur. After retiring from the world of professional fitness modelling in 2015, he now does ultra-endurance events all around the world. In April 2018, he ran the famous Marathon des Sables, which entails six self-sufficient back-to-back marathons through the Sahara Desert in Morocco. In February 2019, he ran 230 km through the Arctic Circle in the northern most tip of Sweden. He documents all his adventures on his social media channels.

After spending more than five years in California and London, Brian currently resides in the West of Ireland, close to where he grew up, with his daughter Holly.

🌐 https://briankeanefitness.com/
🎙 https://briankeanefitness.com/podcast/
📷 www.instagram.com/brian_keane_fitness/?hl=en